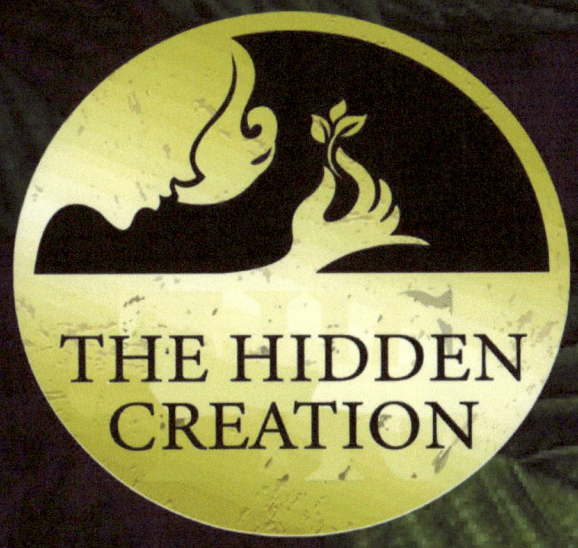

THE HIDDEN CREATION RECIPE BOOK

COOK WITH CANNABIS LIKE A PRO
SAVOR HIDDEN CREATIONS
DIGEST THE HIGH LIFE

VOLUME 1

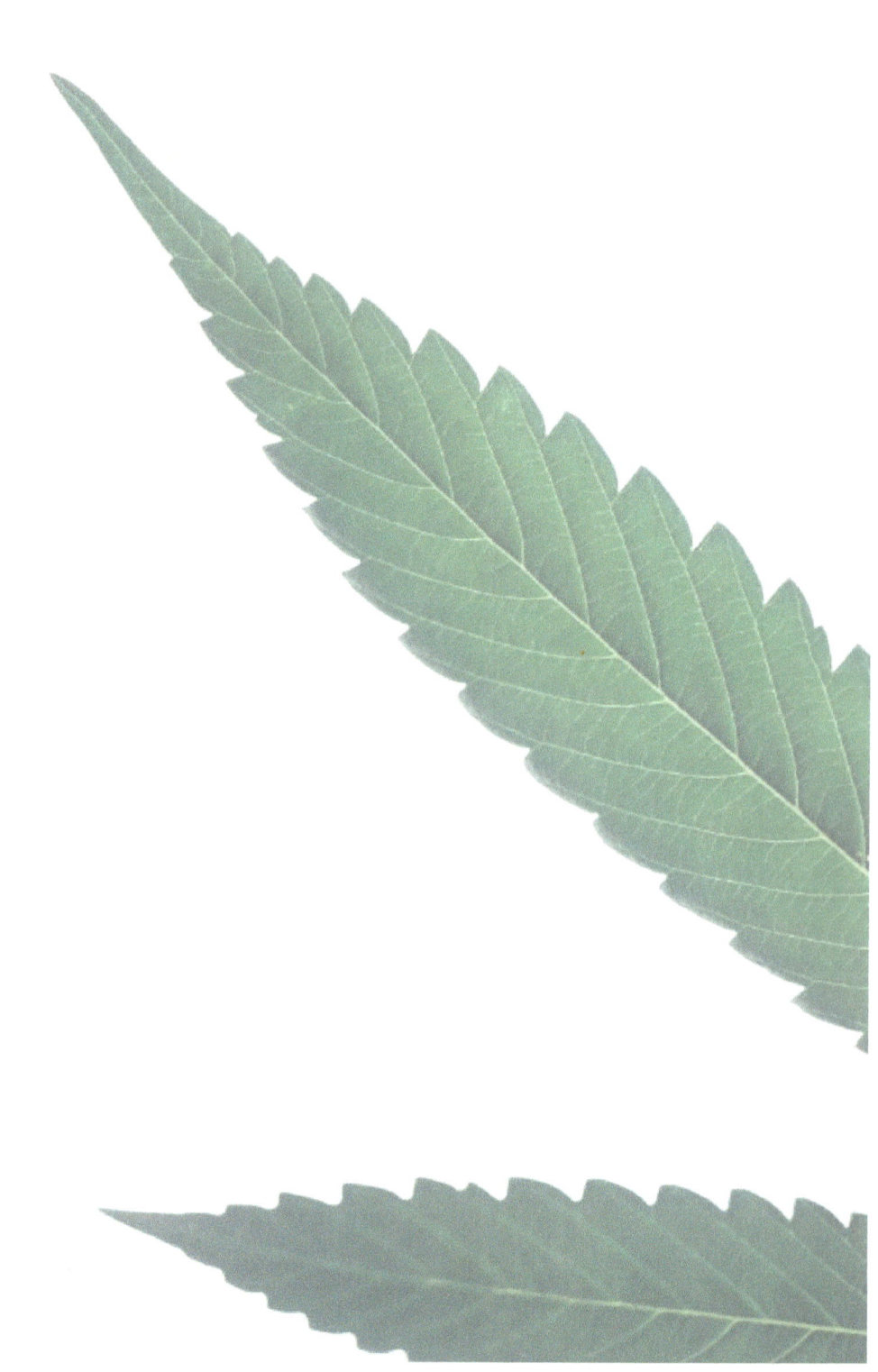

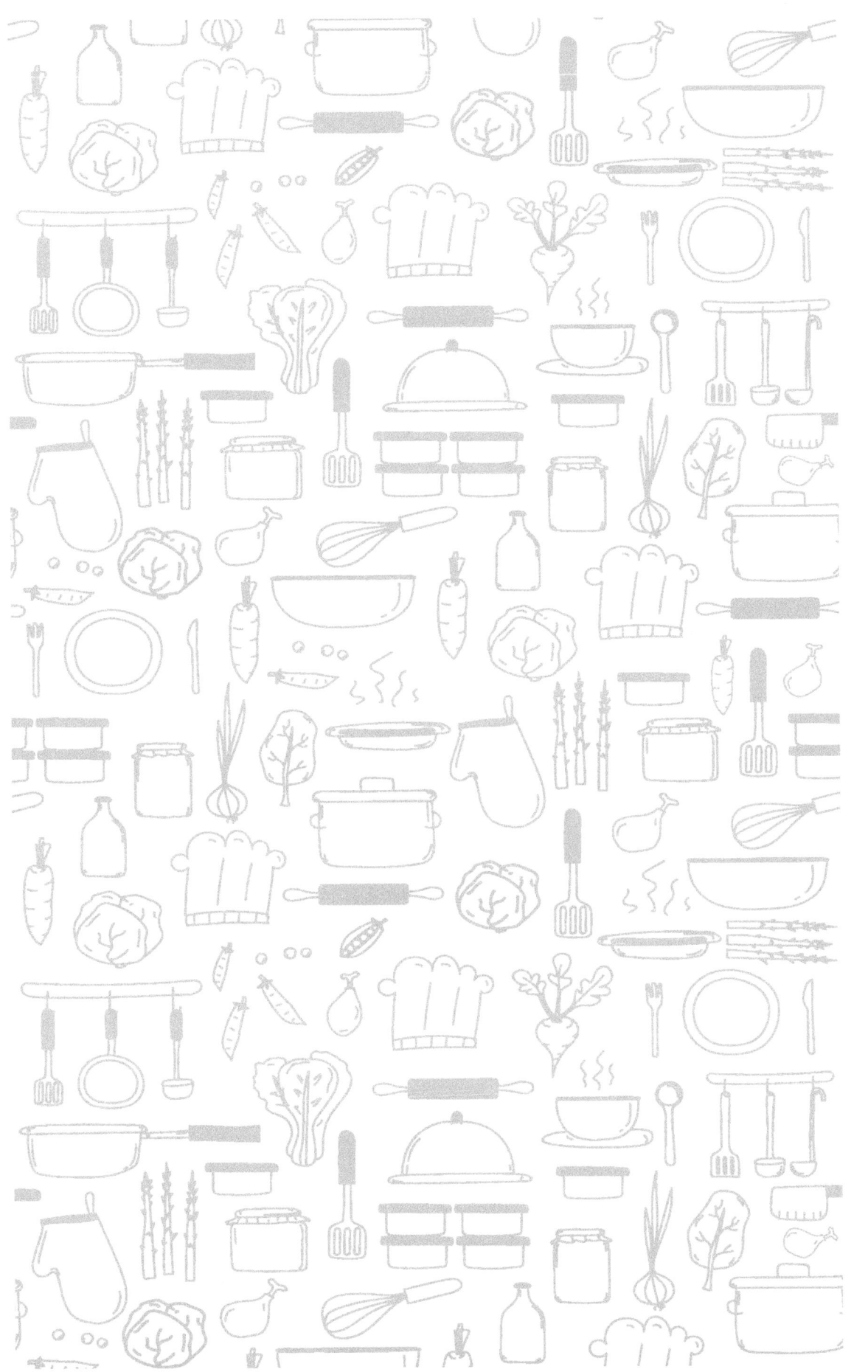

To our first born,

We hope to have made you proud to call us your parents. Your presence has been one of the driving forces behind our journey, and this book stands as a genuine testament to our unwavering perseverance, dedication, determination, and resilience.

COPYRIGHTS

Copyright 2023
by the owners at The Hidden Creation, LLC

All rights reserved. No part of this book may be reproduced or transmitted in any manner whatsoever without written permission from the publisher, except in the case of brief quotations embodied in critical articles or reviews.

Names: The Hidden Creation, LLC

Title: The Hidden Creation Recipe Book: Cook With Cannabis Like A Pro, Savor Hidden Creations, Digest The High Life, Volume 1 / the editors at The Hidden Creation

Description: Miami, Florida : The Hidden Creation 2023

Subjects: Cooking with Cannabis, Recipes, Terminology, Instructions, Conversions, Substitutions, etc.

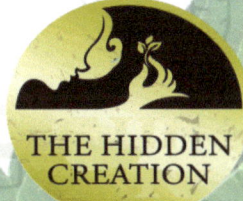

The Hidden Creation, LLC

Miami, Florida

Distributed by The Hidden Creation, LLC
Manufactured in the United States of America

Pictured on front cover: Cannabis Leaf via free ShutterStock images

Author & Editor: Annmarie Sparks

Photographer & Editor : Tarik Sparks

Producers: Annmarie Sparks & Tarik Sparks

Owners of The Hidden Creation, LLC: Tarik & Annmarie Sparks

Other Photo Content: With premissions from Canva.com

Table of Contents

1	**Introduction**
3	**Kitchen Knowledge**
14	**Cannabis Knowledge**
31	**Infusion Methods For Dosing W/Cannabis**
40	**Breads And Doughs**
54	**Soups And Salads**
59	**Appetizers**
65	**Side Dishes**
70	**Main Dishes**
76	**Desserts**
83	**Cannabis Cocktails**
88	**Outro**

Introduction

In the pages of our recipe book, you'll discover a collection of straightforward recipes that make simple to incorporate cannabis into your daily cooking. Whether it's breakfast, lunch, or dinner, we've got you covered with practical, step-by-st instructions.

But this book goes beyond mere recipes. It's an invitation to embark on a culinary adventure. W want you to not only follow our lead but to experiment, innovate, and create your own elevated dining experiences. We've included our best cooking and baking tips to ensure your success in the kitchen.

Moreover, we'll provide you with valuable insights into cannabis – from understanding the different strains to dosage considerations and safety guidelines. Our goal is to equip you with the knowledge you need to navigate the world o cannabis-infused cuisine confidently.

So, whether you're a seasoned chef or a novice i the kitchen, our recipe book is designed to empower you to enjoy the art of cooking with cannabis and create memorable, flavorful moments that you, your family, and friends will cherish.

In this book you will learn:

- 101 Kitchen & Cannabis Fundamentals
- Some Specialty Kitchen Ingredients
- Kitchen Tools We Use Everyday
- Appliances We Love & Need
- Cookware/Bakeware We Can't Live Without
- Substitutions For Meals
- Vegan Alternatives
- Cannabis Language/Knowledge
- Infusion Methods For Dosing w/Cannabis
- Savory Culinary Recipes
- Satisfying Dessert Recipes
- Infused Cannabis Mocktail Recipes
- Recipe Variations
- How To Use Our Cannabis Products
- How To Become A Cannabis Chef
- Who We Are & The Knowledge We Offer
- Upgrade Your Overall Kitchen Skill Set

But this book offers more than just cannabis-infused cuisine. It serves as your gateway to a broader culinary journey, where you'll not only discover how we incorporate cannabis into our dishes but also learn how to craft your own elevated dining experiences.

We're excited to share our favorite insights, essential cannabis knowledge, and key points to ensure you're well-equipped to embark on this flavorful ground-breaking adventure.

Kitchen Knowledge

17	**Conversions & Equivalents**
18	**Cookware/Bakeware**
19	**Kitchen Appliances**
20	**Kitchen Tools**
21	**Specialty Ingredients**
22	**Substitutions/Allergens**

This section outlines the kitchen items you'll need to effortlessly follow our recipes. Within this chapter, we've also included references for ingredient substitutions and conversions.

If you have any dietary restrictions, be sure to bookmark this chapter. It will allow you to adjust each of our recipes to meet your specific needs.

Conversions & Equivalents

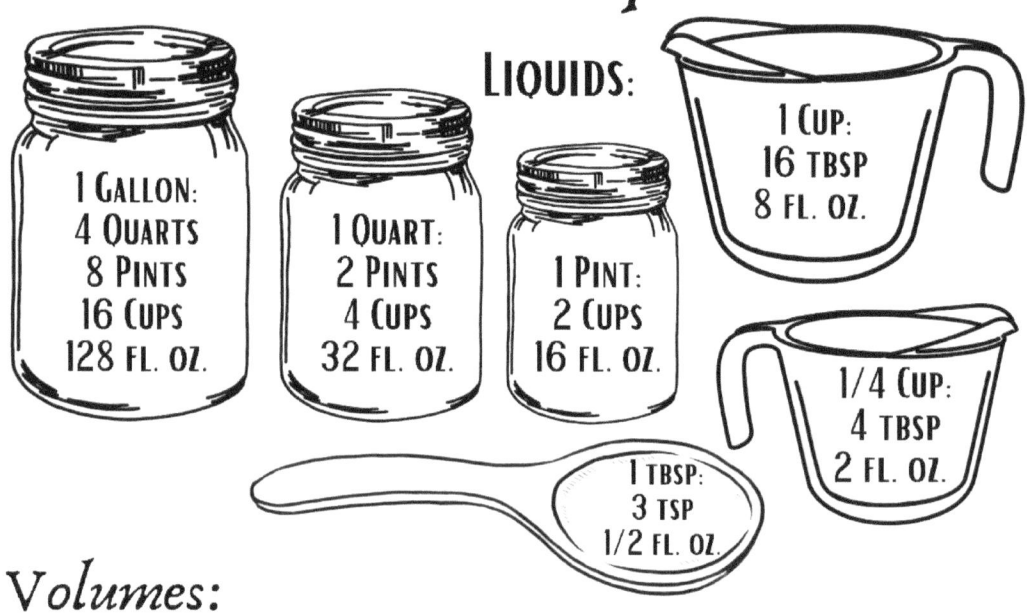

Liquids:

- 1 Gallon: 4 Quarts, 8 Pints, 16 Cups, 128 Fl. Oz.
- 1 Quart: 2 Pints, 4 Cups, 32 Fl. Oz.
- 1 Pint: 2 Cups, 16 Fl. Oz.
- 1 Cup: 16 Tbsp, 8 Fl. Oz.
- 1/4 Cup: 4 Tbsp, 2 Fl. Oz.
- 1 Tbsp: 3 Tsp, 1/2 Fl. Oz.

Volumes:

Fluid Oz.	Teaspoons	Tablespoons	Cups	Liters
1/2 Fl. Oz.	3 Tsp.	1 Tbsp.	1/16 cup	15 mL
1 Fl. Oz.	6 Tsp.	2 Tbsp.	1/8 cup	30 mL
2 Fl. Oz.	12 Tsp.	4 Tbsp.	1/4 cup	60 mL
2.7 Fl. Oz.	16 Tsp.	5 & 1/3 Tbsp.	1/3 cup	80 mL
4 Fl. Oz.	24 Tsp.	8 Tbsp.	1/2 cup	120 mL
6 Fl. Oz.	36 Tsp.	12 Tbsp.	3/4 cup	180 mL
8 Fl. Oz.	48 Tsp.	16 Tbsp.	1 cup	240 mL

Some measurements have been rounded for ease of use.

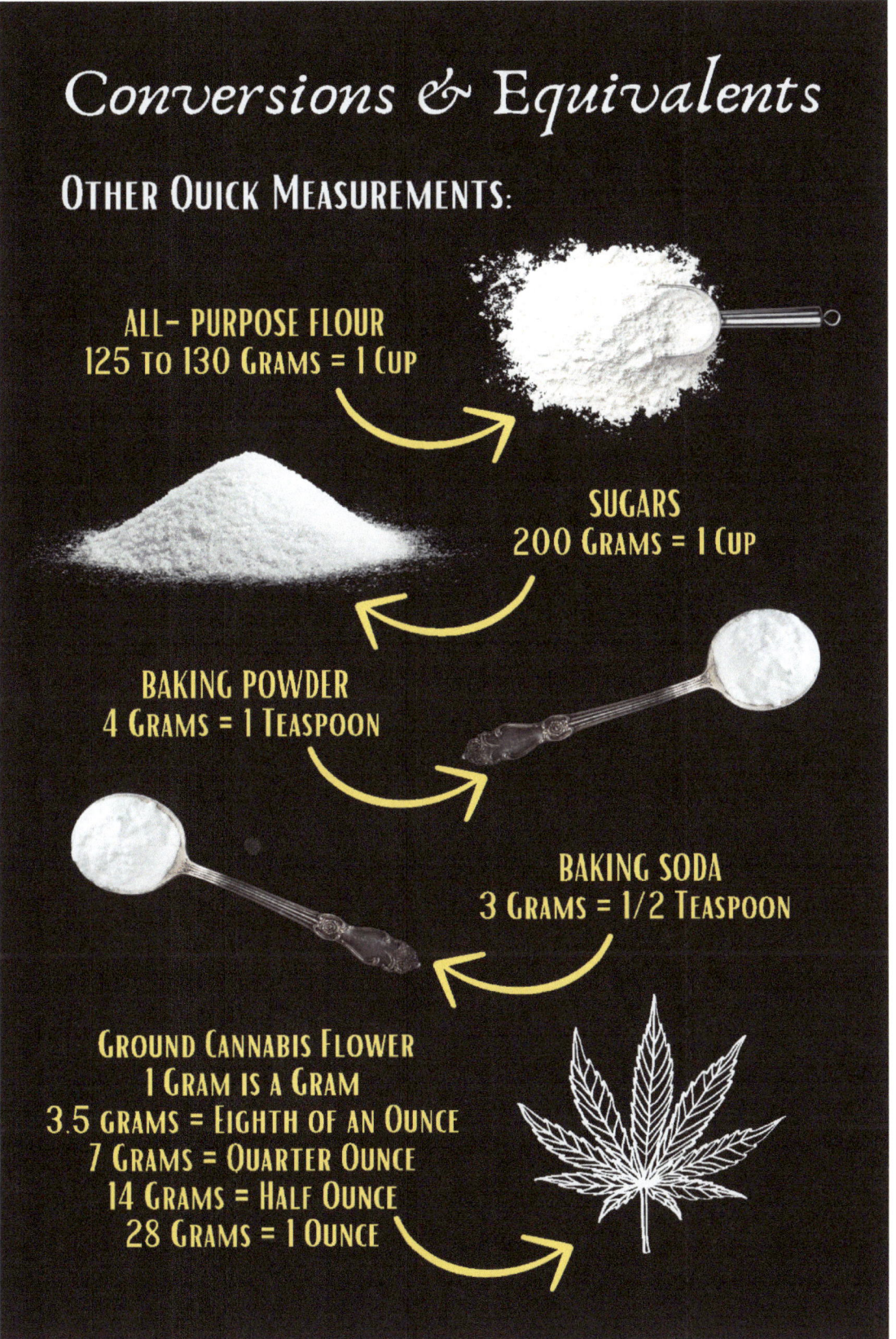

Conversions & Equivalents

More Quick Measurements:

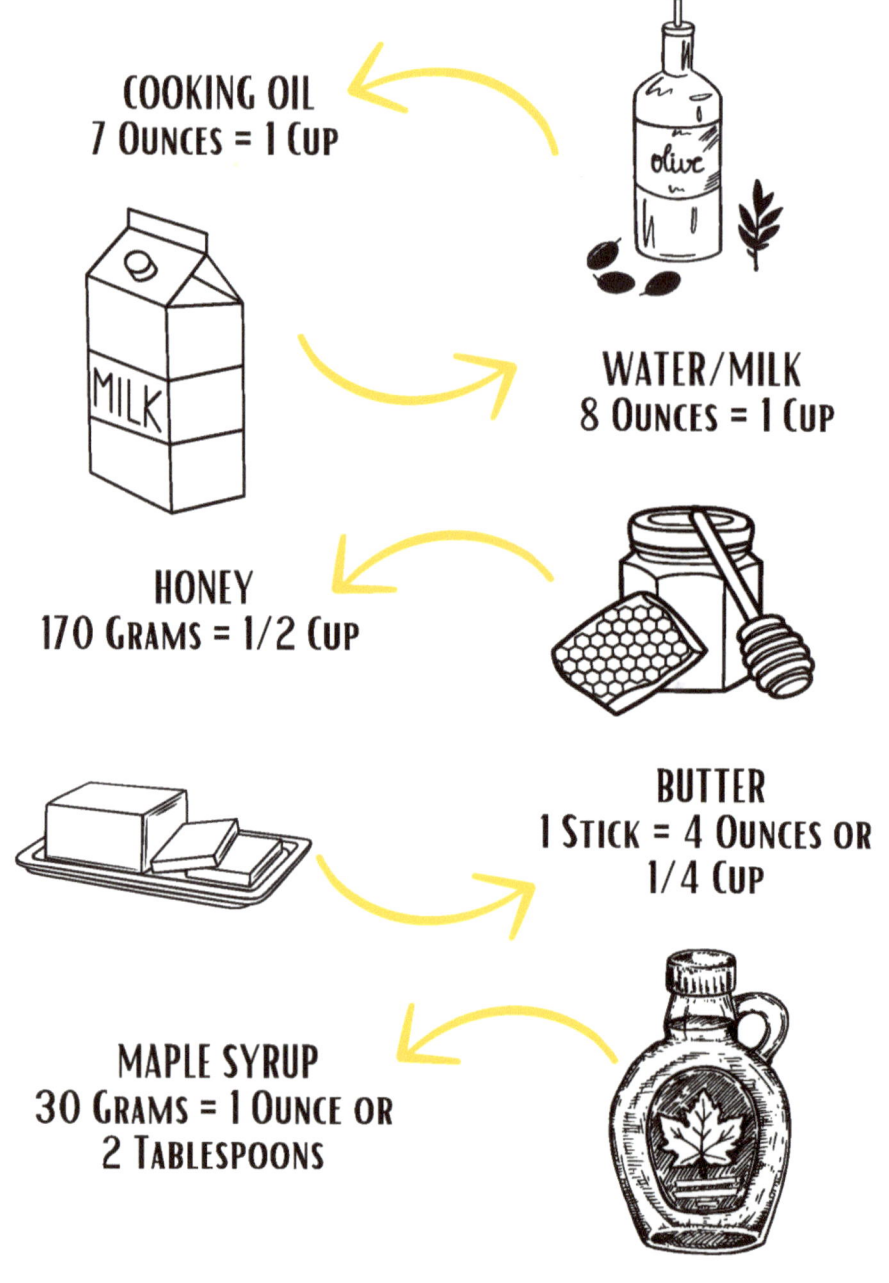

COOKING OIL
7 Ounces = 1 Cup

WATER/MILK
8 Ounces = 1 Cup

HONEY
170 Grams = 1/2 Cup

BUTTER
1 Stick = 4 Ounces or 1/4 Cup

MAPLE SYRUP
30 Grams = 1 Ounce or 2 Tablespoons

Cookware / Bakeware

Here are additional kitchen essentials necessary for preparing recipes from our book, or any cookbook for that matter. There's no need for detailed explanations as you may already have these items:

- **Baking Pans**
- **Cast Iron Pans**
- **Cooling Racks**
- **Cupcake Pan**
- **Dutch Oven**
- **Frying Pan**
- **Glass Baking Pans**
- **Large Stock Pot**
- **Loaf Pan**
- **Non-Stick Pizza Pan**
- **Sauce Pot**
- **Sauté Pan**
- **Sheet Pans**

No need to worry. If you don't have many of these items, you can still proceed with simpl substitutes. For instance, if you don't have a Dutch Oven, a regular large pot will do the jo just note it won't be the same. (Like a B.L.T. with no bacon... just not the same - sadly, people still order their sandwiches this way...)

Kitchen Appliances

To cook with purpose, you'll need the proper machinery. To infuse like a professional, you'll need the right machinery. You literally need the right kitchen appliance to do what we do. No shortcuts. We literally have no clu of what's in your kitchen so take a look at every applianc we have in ours and why we use them:

Ardent FX Decarboxylator
This machine is an excellent investment for your home kitchen. It not only decarboxylates your cannabis but also infuses it, and you can even bake in it. The other well-known brands include Magic Butter Machine and Levo Oil Infuser.

Countertop Stand Blender
This refers to your Vitamix or cheaper counterpart, which is great for blending large amounts of liquids or purees at a time without making a huge mess.

Food Grade Dehydrator
We can be a bit fancy at times, so this machine is perfect for drying out fruits, vegetables, and so much more. Substitute this item by turning your oven on the lowest setting, adding your items to a sheet tray lined with parchment paper and a few hours of patience.

Juicer
This was all the rage, and we wanted one. We rarely use it, but when we do, we absolutely love it. Just imagine fresh juices for stocks, marinating/brining different foods, and all the wonderful homemade juices. This one's definitely now a requirement. You can easily use cheesecloth paired with a strainer after blending. (For example: if you want strawberry juice, blend the item first with additional liquid and double strain after to expel all of the unwanted fruit fragments.

KitchenAid Stand Mixer
This is our everything. As you can imagine, there are countless possibilities with one of these. These are a little pricey but you can usually get these on a great clearance some where if you look for it. Otherwise, get another brand name or knockoff that works for you.

KitchenAid Pasta Attachment
Because making pasta from scratch is life. However, there are many ways to create pasta shapes without it. There are endless pasta video tutorials on this. Of course, you don't need this versio or brand. There are plenty of pasta makers to choose from.

Kitchen Scale
Most recommended as we do not usually measure in cups. If you do not own a scale or just prefer cup measurements, please use google to convert the recipe or refer to our "Equivalents & Conversions" section in this book to guide you.

Hand Emulsion Blender
Some sauces and/or stocks benefit from having one of these hand in your kitchen. They're pretty inexpensive and we highly recommend owning one of these. With this item you may even get away with not having a Magic Bullet. With a little patience you can substitute this for. Stand mixer and food processor as well. All in all, don't skip owning one of these.

Magic Bullet Personal Sized Blender
If you do not own a hand blender, this is also great to have. We use this especially to make sauces like pesto, chimichurri, salsa, etc.

Mandolin & Peeler
Naturally, we prefer a mandolin, this is the most efficient way to slice all of your fruits and vegetables evenly. Even cuts makes for even cooking. A peeler can be substituted for a small pairing knife but honestly just buy the peeler.

Robot Coupe aka Food Processor
This baby does it all from chopping vegetables to pureeing sweet potatoes to making pasta dough and if you spend a little extra, it w have additional attachment to shred cheese in half the time.

Spice Grinder
This is a must buy, you will thank us later! If you don't want to grind up your black pepper by hand, buy this. If you want to grind your cannabis in larger quantities, buy this. The best part is, coffee grinders are usually cheaper and still works like a charm. We own of these!

Small Scale
For weighing lighter/smaller amounts. You need to be able to accurately scale your bud and/or ingredients like yeast or small liquid amounts in grams. In some cases you can use a teaspoon/tablespoon set (for this, also refer to our "Equivalents & Conversions" section in this book to guide you.)

And of course a:
Freezer, Microwave, Oven, Refrigerator & Stove Top (a gas stove is superior if you have it)

Kitchen Tools

As chefs we hold our kitchen tools very close to our hearts just as any chef at any restaurant never goes to work without their knife bag. Your kitchen tools ar what makes cooking in the kitchen a breeze. Here ar our must-haves & why:

Can Opener
A hand held opener works fine and the electric ones are also great. You may also want the little one that punctures triangle holes on the top of the can for milk.

Chef's Knife
No way around this. You'll need a good quality chefs knife for just about everything knife related.

Citrus Squeezer
For a quick lemon, lime or orange juice squeeze when you only need smaller amounts.

Cooking Spatula
For flipping just about anything that needs to be flipped or lifting food that need to be lifted.

Cooking Spoon
Used for cooking, stirring, basting, transferring food and serving.

Cutting Board
This is very self explanatory but if you don't have one, you should get one.

Kitchen Scissors
Also self explanatory. You have to be able to open things that need to be opened. Of course you can just use a knife too.

Mixing Bowls
Great for marinating, mixing and so many other basic needs for having a bowl.

Offset Spatula
Not absolutely essential but it makes spreading anything out much easier.

Pairing Knife
For small incisions or cuts. Use for cutting small fruits/vegetables, etc.

Peeler
For peeling fruits or vegetables..

Pyrex Glass Measuring Cups
Use this for liquids you need to measure, blend, warm up or put to the side.

Rolling Pin
You'll need this for rolling out different doughs

Rubber Mixing Spatula
We do not waste anything, so these in abundance are great for mixing ingredients well and scraping it all out.

Serrated Knife
For cutting breads, certain types of large fruit, cake, etc.

Tasting Spoons
Because they're tiny and cute which makes them great for tasting your food and stirring your honey into your tea.

Thermometer
For accurately cooking food to the proper temperature.

Tongs
Great for picking up hot food, flipping food and moving food around.

Whisk
A good sturdy whisk is great for quick mixing. Don't buy a flimsy one just becasue it's cute.

Specialty Ingredients

We know everyone shops differently, but please have an open mind to try something new with us. Some of these items may b familiar to you and some may not. Different sugars do taste/react different in each recipe. And vanilla bean matters!

Truffle Oil
Try this if you're feeling fancy enough to elevate your taste buds.

Fresh Cracked Black Pepper
Because its better - don't be lazy.

Coarse Kosher Salt
Please throw away any & all iodine salt. Try Himalayan pink salt or sea salt instead. Or shop specialty salts at your local farmers market.

Fresh Herbs
The more the merrier - they're great!

Mushrooms
We do not use white mushrooms in our kitchen - no flavor. Try shitake, portabella, porcini, oyster mushrooms instead.

Nutritional Yeast
is a deactivated yeast also known as hippy dust. It's a staple in our kitchen and is great for adding a natural cheesy flavor.

All-Purpose Flour
We only use King Author's flour. It's literally the crème de la crème. Google it!

Sugar
We love all sugar but specifically rich in flavor kinds like: cane sugar & dark brown sugar. It's not healthier but trust the flavor speaks for itself.

Unsalted Butter
It is so much better to add the salt in yourself, this way you can control the salt content. Use non-dairy butter in lieu if that's your preference (just bare in mind, this won't harden back up in the refrigerator the same once it's been melted).

Vanilla
Get yourself some quality Madagascar vanilla bean paste, extract and/or fresh pods. Please do not buy imitation anything!

Yeast
Essential for awesome bread making. Yeast comes in 3 varieties: fresh, active & instant. Most of our recipes will call for active yeast.

Substitutions / Allergens

These are great alternatives for the upcoming recipes whether it be for dietary restrictions or just not having any of that particular ingredient. We consider ourselves to be flexitarian which to us means that we are more health conscious about what we consume without always giving up the food we enjoy.

Crustaceans/ Fish/ Mollusk
If you have a shellfish or seafood allergy, you can switch these items out for anything else you would prefer in its place for any recipe. There are many vegan alternatives that you can buy in-store or online.

Coconut
We love coconut as a replacement for heavy cream for our alfredo pasta or any creamy white sauce.

Dairy
We love cheese! Very interchangeably we will use vegan, non-vega or homemade cheese alternatives. As far as everything else containing dairy, we prefer it vegan. Feel free to use whatever works for you!

Eggs
We use eggs but we also interchangeably use a vegan alternative by Bob's Red Mill and its fantastic for baking substitutions.

Gluten/ Wheat
If you did not know, most soy products do contain gluten. Either avoid soy all-together or find items that show that they are gluten-free soy options. As for flour, try using King Authors Gluten-Free Flour Mix the way they recommend doing so.

Peanuts
Very rarely do we ever cook with peanuts but if you're having a meal like pad Thai, pine nuts (if you're not allergic to them) are a great substitute.

Tree Nuts
If you're allergic, obviously don't use it or replace with an alternative like your favorite kind of seeds.

Cannabis Knowledge

19	**Cannabinoids**
24	**Cannabis Terminology**
26	**Cannabis Terpenes**
32	**Endocannabinoid System**
33	**Methods of Administration**

On the other hand, it's one thing to love cannabis but it's another world to fully understand it's language. Undoubtly, this is the most important chapter of this book.

After all, without it, you just have a plain ole-basic-everybody-anybody-can do it recipe book.

Cannabinoids

What are cannabinoids?

Cannabinoids are a group of chemical compounds found in the cannabis plant and produced naturally by the human body. They interact with the body's endocannabinoid system, a vital internal regulatory system that regulates functions like pain sensation, immune response, mood, appetite, and memory. The endocannabinoid system comprises CB1 and CB2 receptors, found throughout the body, and cannabinoids, which bind to these receptors to produce various effects.

The two most well-known cannabinoids are tetrahydrocannabinol (THC) and cannabidiol (CBD). THC is the primary psychoactive component of cannabis and causes the "high" commonly associated with marijuana use. CBD, conversely, does not have psychoactive effects and is being studied for potential therapeuti benefits, such as reducing anxiety and inflammation. Cannabis contains a numerous amount of other cannabinoids, each with unique properties and potential benefits.

What does this mean for us?

Currently, scientists have identified over 200 distinct cannabinoid in cannabis, with the potential for more, as there are over 750 natural chemical components of the plant yet to be fully researched. Each of these compounds has a unique effect on the endocannabinoid system.

Common Therapeutic Effects:

Aids Sleep: CBN
Anti-Anxiety: CBD
Anti-Inflammatory: CBC, CBD, CBG, CBN, THCA
Anti-Depressant: CBD, THC
Anti-Nausea: CBD, THC
Anti-Oxidant: CBD, THC
Appetite Stimulant: THC
Relieves Pain: CBC, CBD, CBN, THC

Let's take a look at some of the most common cannabinoids found. On the next few pages you'll recognize some of your favorites, some you've vaguely heard of and others that may not seem so common to you. Cannabinoids ending in "A" most likely refers to th acidic form of the cannabinoid. We will explain the acidic form of THC. This section of the book is a great reference if you're looking for a specific cannabinoid to infuse your meals with.

CBC

CBC is a non-psychoactive cannabinoid found in the cannabis plant. It has potential therapeutic benefits such as anti-inflammatory and pain-relieving properties, and may promote neurogenesis. CBC interacts with the body's endocannabinoid system by binding to CB2 receptors primarily found in immune cells and the peripheral nervous system. It is a promising area of research in cannabinoid science.

CBD

CBD, or cannabidiol, is a naturally occurring compound found in the cannabis plant. It is one of many cannabinoids found in the plant and is known for its potential therapeutic effects, including reducing anxiety, pain, and inflammation. CBD does not produce the psychoactive effects associated with THC, another cannabinoid found in cannabis. It is also important to note that CBD is most widely known for significantly reducing seizures in epileptic patient among other neuro pathic disorders and conditions.

CBDA

CBDA, or cannabidiolic acid, is a non-psychoactive cannabinoid found in raw, unheated cannabis plants. It is the acidic precursor to CBD and is converted to CBD through a process called decarboxylation, which occurs when the plant is heated or exposed to sunlight.

CBG

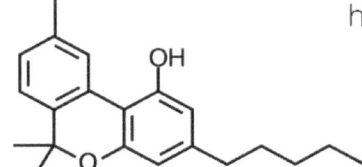

CBG, or cannabigerol, is another cannabinoid found in the cannabis plant. It is often referred to as the "stem cell" or "mother" cannabinoid, as it is a precursor to many other cannabinoids, including THC and CBD. CBG has been the subject of research for its potential therapeutic effects, including reducing inflammation and pain, and it may also have antibacterial and neuroprotective properties. However, more research is needed to fully understand its effects on human health.

CBN

Cannabinol (CBN) is a minor cannabinoid found in the cannabis plant. It is produced from the degradation of tetrahydrocannabinol (THC), which occurs over time as the plant ages or when exposed to heat or light. CBN is believed to have mild psychoactive properties, but it is much less potent than THC.

CBN has been studied for its potential therapeutic benefits, including its ability to promote sleep and relieve pain. It is als believed to have antibacterial and anti-inflammatory properties, and to be a potent appetite stimulant. However, much more research is needed to fully understand the effect of CBN and its potential applications.

DELTA 8

Delta-8-tetrahydrocannabinol (delta-8 or D8) is a minor cannabinoid that occurs naturally in cannabis in very small amounts. It is structurally similar to delta-9-tetrahydrocannabinol (delta-9 or THC), the primary psychoactive compound found in cannabis, but it has a slightly different chemical structure. Delta-8 is known for producing a milder high than delta-9, with fewer adverse effects such as anxiety and paranoia. Delta-8 has been the subject of recent interest as a potential therapeutic compound, but more research is needed to fully understand its effects on human health. Delta-8 is often derived from hemp and may be legal under certain circumstances, but its legality can vary depending on local laws and regulations.

DELTA 10

Delta-10-tetrahydrocannabinol (delta-10 or D10) is a rare and relatively new cannabinoid that has been identified in some cannabis strains. It is structurally similar to delta-9-tetrahydrocannabinol (delta-9 or THC) and delta-8-tetrahydrocannabinol (delta-8 or D8), but it has a slightly different chemical structure.

Delta-10 is believed to have psychoactive effects similar to those of delta-9 and delta-8, but research on its effects is limited. Delta-10 is not present in significant quantities in mos cannabis strains, and it is typically produced by converting other cannabinoids, such as CBD or delta-9, using chemical processes. The legal status of delta-10 can vary depending on local laws and regulations, and it may not be legal in all jurisdictions.

THC

THC, or delta-9-tetrahydrocannabinol, is the primary psychoactive compound found in the cannabis plant. It is the chemical responsible for producing the characteristic "high" or euphoric effects associated with cannabis use. THC works by binding to cannabinoid receptors in the brain, which can affect mood, perception, and cognition. THC also has potential therapeutic properties, including pain relief, nausea reduction, and appetite stimulation. However, THC can also have adverse effects, such as anxiety, paranoia, and impaired coordination, especially when consumed in high doses.

THCA

THCA, or tetrahydrocannabinolic acid, is a non-psychoactive cannabinoid that is found in raw and live cannabis plants. When heated or aged, THCA is converted to THC, which is the psychoactive compound that is associated with the "high" commonly associated with cannabis. THCA is being studied for its potential therapeutic effects, which may include anti-inflammatory, neuroprotective, and anti-emetic properties.

THCV

THCV is a cannabinoid found in the cannabis plant that has unique effects compared to THC. It may suppress appetite, have neuroprotective properties, and potential in the treatment of neurological disorders. THCV interacts with CB1 and CB2 receptors but has weaker binding affinity than THC. Further research is needed to fully understand its therapeuti potential.

Cannabis Terminology

All of this cannabis talk can be a lot to take in, so we hope this helps.

Cannabinoids are chemical compounds which act on cannabinoid receptors. There are 3 types of cannabinoids compounds: endocanbabinoids, phytocannabinoids & synthetic cannabinoids. The most common known types today are THC & CBD from the phytocannabinoid family.

Cannabis is also known as flower, marijuana, bud, etc.

CBD is the abbreviation for cannabidiol is the second most known cannabinoid. CBD has recently gained attention for its use as a medical treatment as research has shown it effectively treats pain, inflammation and anxiety, without the psychoactive effects (the "high" or "stoned" feeling) associated with THC.

Decarboxylate is a chemical reaction that uses heat and time to remove a carboxyl group (a.k.a. the acidic form) from cannabinoids in the cannabis plant, enhancing their ability to interact with your body's receptors (a.k.a. the way you get medicated)

Distillate is a type of concentrate that is created through a extensive distillation process that separates other compounds from cannabis plant matter leaving a runny, translucent oil devoid of the waxes or undesirable compounds from the original plant.

Endocannabinoids are neurotransmitters produced by human tissue.

Hybrid refers to a plant that is genetically a cross between one or more separate strains of cannabis. Most marijuana found on the market today is some form of hybrid.

Indica is the less scientific name that basically means it tends to produce more relaxing physical effects and can have sedative qualities because it binds to your CB2 rceptors which are more widely spread in the body.

Isolate is a crystalline solid or powder that is 99% pure. The extraction process removes all the active compounds from the cannabis plant and then it is refined to contain only contain one type of cannabinoid.

Kief is a collected amount of trichomes that have been separated from the rest of the marijuana flower. Since trichomes are the sticky crystals that contain the vast majority of the plant's cannabinoids, kief is known to be extremely potent.

Phytocannabinoids are naturally occurring cannabinoids found in plants. More than 100 cannabinoids have been identified in the hemp plant.

RSO (also known as Rick Simpson Oil) is an odorless and viscous cannabis concentrate that's densely packed with phytocannabinoids from a process that cooks the cannabis in a high proof alcohol that is then reduced.

Sativa is the less scientific name that basically means it tends to produce more cerebral effects as opposed to physical and sedative ones because it binds to your CB1 receptors.

Synthetic Cannabinoids are self explanatory... these are man made.

Terpenes are responsible for the aroma and flavors of cannabis. It also influences effects by interacting with cannabinoids.

THC is short for tetrahydrocannabinol a.k.a. delta-9. It is the most well-known and most abundantly available cannabinoid in marijuana plants. THC is also the component in marijuana that is responsible for the psychoactive effects, or the "high." There are new emerging THC cannabinoids still being found including the very recent Delta 8 THC cannabinoid which is similar but has less effects.

Tincture is a liquid cannabis extract usually made with alcohol, MCT oil or glycerol that is often dosed in a dropper bottle. Tinctures can be flavored and are usually placed under the tongue, where they are absorbed quickly.

Trichomes are the little fibers that grow from the cannabis plant (a.k.a. the really pretty part to observe with a magnifying glass).

Wax/Crumble refers to a potent cannabis concentrate that has been agitated during the extraction process, causing the oil to crystallize and solidify. The consistency and texture of wax can range from gooey or creamy to something harder and flaky, known as crumble or honeycomb. Higher-quality waxes tend to be softer and amber-toned.

Cannabis Terpenes

Terpenes are organic compounds found in the trichomes of female cannabis plants that produce distinctive aromas, enrich color and pigmentation in leaves and buds, and contribute to the flavor of cannabis.

Terpenes help to enhance the plant's attractiveness to some creatures while deterring others that can do harm. The amount o terpenes a cannabis plant produces can be affected by variables like the growing conditions, temperature, nutrient levels, and harvest time.

The effects of terpenes extend beyond feel-good benefits and stress relief, with many boasting unique combinations of therapeutic properties such as antiviral, anticancer,antidepressant , and antimicrobial activity.

Some terpenes are volatile compounds, which can be easily lost during cannabis extraction processes, but methods such as live resin that maintain freezing temperatures throughout the extraction process can protect terpenes and other volatile compounds in the plant.

The 5 most common terpenes found include: Caryophylene, Humulene, Limonene, Myrcene and Pinene.

The beauty in terpenes is that they are not just found in cannabis but in everyday natural resources. You'll recognize some of the names and realize that you've already been introducing terpenes into your lifestyle. There are many terpenes known to date and we 'll cover some of the most common sought after as well as a few others you may or may not have already heard of.

From the section of the book, our biggest take away is that when you're sourcing your cannabis to infuse your meal with, take a second learn about the strain you're working with. Maybe you don 't need a strain that's going to make you relaxed because of the Myrcene terpene found in it. Maybe instead you're looking for a strain to aid with anxiety or pain relief.

Beyond flavor profile of food and aromas of the strain you choose, infuse with purpose. We guarantee you'll surprise yourself as well as your peers!

BISABOLOL

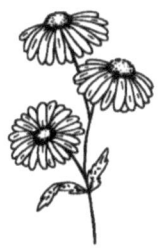

Aromas/Flavors:
warm floral nutty fruity aroma with herbal peppery undertones
Therapeutic Effects:
anti-inflammatory, anti-microbial, anti-biotic, anti-oxidant, anti-cancer, anti-anxiety, anti-depression & analgesic properties
Also Found In:
chamomile, candeia tree, sage & cannabis

BORNEOL

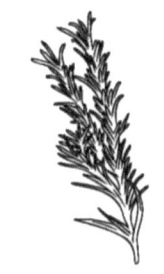

Aromas/Flavors:
cool minty spicy scent
Therapeutic Effects:
anti-inflammatory, neuroprotective, anesthetic & anti-oxidant properties
Also Found In:
ginger, rosemary, camphor, thyme & cannabis

CAMPHENE

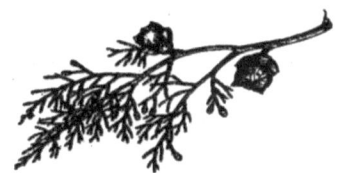

Aromas/Flavors:
pungent, strong aroma reminiscent of wet pine needles on a forest floor like "wet earth"
Therapeutic Effects:
therapeutic properties with anti-microbial, anti-viral, pain-relieving effects & can provide cough relief
Also Found In:
nutmeg, cypress oil, bergamot oil, camphor oil, moth balls, valerian & cannabis

CAMPHOR

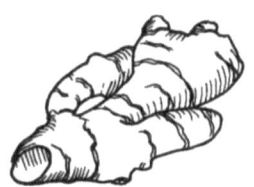

Aromas/Flavors:
strong menthol-like aroma
Therapeutic Effects:
used to treat skin conditions, improve respiratory function, relieve pain, used as an anti-bacterial, anti-fungal & has anti-inflammatory properties
Also Found In:
spiced fruit, vegetables and herbs such as raspberry, apricot, ginger & cannabis

B-CARYOPHYLLENE

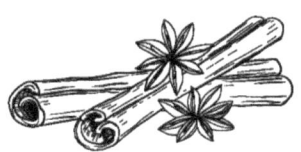

Aromas/Flavors:
slight bite of pungency associated with smelling cracked pepper

Therapeutic Effects:
anti-inflammatory, pain relief, anti-bacterial, anti-oxidant, anti-anxiety, anti-depression & treating inflammatory bowel disease

Also Found In:
basil, copaiba, black caraway, oregano, lavender, allspice, fig, roman chamomile, cloves, hops, cinnamon, ylang-ylang, rosemary & cannabis

GERANIOL

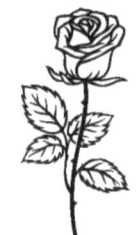

Aromas/Flavors:
sweet delicate rose & floral profile

Therapeutic Effects:
anti-oxidant, anti-inflammatory, neuro-protective & anti-depressant

Also Found In:
rose oil, lemongrass, lemons, peaches, grapefruits, oranges, carrots, coriander, blueberries, blackberries & cannabis

EUCALYPTOL

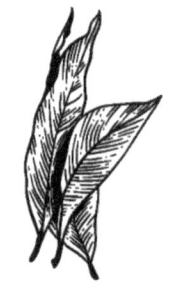

Aromas/Flavors:
fresh, mint-like with spicy, cooling taste

Therapeutic Effects:
pain-relieving, anti-bacterial, anti-fungal, anti-inflammatory, anti-proliferative, anti-oxidant

Also Found In:
eucalyptus trees, bay leaves, cardamom, tea tree, sage & cannabis

HUMULENE

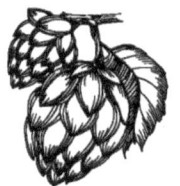

Aromas/Flavors:
earthy, woody, with spicy, herbal notes

Therapeutic Effects:
anti-bacterial, anti-allergic, anti-inflammatory, anti-tumor, anti-cancer, as well as relief from insomnia, depression, anxiety & digestive disorders

Also Found In:
hops, basil, cloves, sage & cannabis

LIMONENE

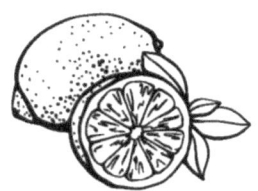

Aromas/Flavors:
a freshly squeezed lemon
Therapeutic Effects:
served to reduce stress, elevate mood, anxiety relief, nausea relief, pain relief, anti-fungal properties, anti-bacterial properties, it may help relieve heartburn & gastric reflux
Also Found In:
lemon rind, rosemary, orange rind, juniper & cannabis

MYRCENE

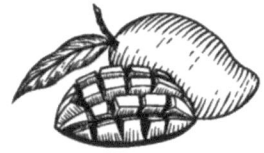

Aromas/Flavors:
earthy, musky notes, resembling cloves with fruity, red grape-like aromas
Therapeutic Effects:
improve sleep, reduce pain, promote relaxation, relieve anxiety & strengthen the immune system
Also Found In:
thyme, mango, lemongrass, hops, houttuynia, myrcia, verbena, West Indian Bay Tree & cannabis

LINALOOL

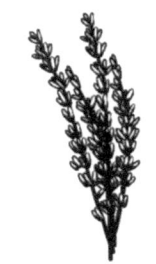

Aromas/Flavors:
sweet floral aroma of lavender scent with a hint of spiciness
Therapeutic Effects:
supports calming effects, relaxation, mood elevation, anti-depressant, anti-microbial, appetite stimulant & anti-anxiety
Also Found In:
ginger, rosemary, camphor, thyme & cannabis

NEROLIDOL

Aromas/Flavors:
faint woody, floral, slightly rose-apple aroma
Therapeutic Effects:
sedative-relaxing effects, aids with sleep, anti-oxidant, anti-fungal, anti-cancer, anti-microbial & anti-parasitic
Also Found In:
jasmine, tea tree, lemongrass, rose, citronella, ginger & cannabis

OCIMENE

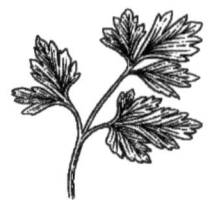

Aromas/Flavors:
sweet, earthy, citrusy aroma frequently used in perfume
Therapeutic Effects:
uplifting effects, anti-convulsant, anti-inflammatory, anti-viral & anti-fungal
Also Found In:
mint, parsley, orchids, hops, kumquats, mangoes, basil, bergamot, lavender, orchids, pepper & cannabis

B-PINENE

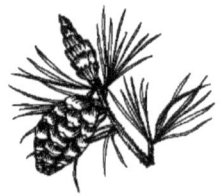

Aromas/Flavors:
fresh, woody, and spicy (similar dill, parsley, basil or hops)
Therapeutic Effects:
pain relief, anti-bacterial, anti-inflammatory, anti-proliferative, anti-oxidant, neuro-generative & bronchodilatotor
Also Found In:
basil, cedar, pine, and conifer trees, dill, eucalyptus, oranges, parsley, rosemary & cannabis

PHYTOL

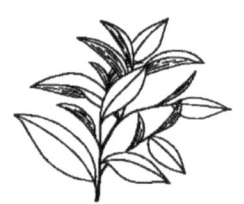

Aromas/Flavors:
grassy and balsamic
Therapeutic Effects:
for reducing inflammation, pain, anxiety, may also be helpful as an anti-oxidant, anti-tumor agent, as well as a sedative & anti-convulsant.
Also Found In:
green tea plants, algae, bacteria & cannabis

A-PINENE

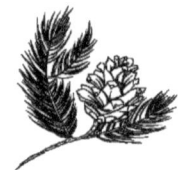

Aromas/Flavors:
fresh and earthy scent (similar to pine & rosemary)
Therapeutic Effects:
pain relief, anti-bacterial, anti-inflammatory, anti-proliferative & anti-oxidant
Also Found In:
pine and conifer trees, rosemary, orange peels & cannabis

SABINENE

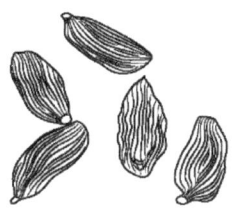

Aromas/Flavors:
citrusy, woody, spicy, peppery
Therapeutic Effects:
anti-inflammatory, anti-fungal, anti-microbial, anti-bacterial & anti-oxidant
Also Found In:
nutmeg, basil, marjoram, cloves, cardamom & cannabis

A-TERPINENE

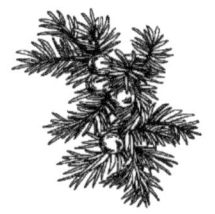

Aromas/Flavors:
smoky & woody
Therapeutic Effects:
anti-bacterial, anti-fungal, anti-insomnia, anti-proliferative & anti-oxidant
Also Found In:
allspice, eucalyptus, citrus, juniper, cardamom, marjoram & cannabis

TERPINEOL

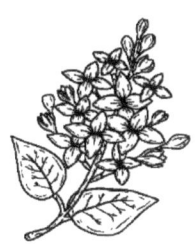

Aromas/Flavors:
fresh lilac, with floral and woody undertones
Therapeutic Effects:
anti-biotic, anti-oxidant, anti-tumor, sedative, anti-inflammatory, anti-malarial & anxiolytic
Also Found In:
lilacs, pine trees, lime blossoms, eucalyptus sap & cannabis

TERPINOLINE

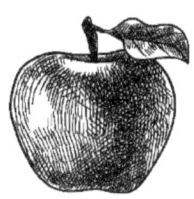

Aromas/Flavors:
smoky, woody, floral, herbal & occasionally citrusy
Therapeutic Effects:
anti-bacterial, anti-fungal, anti-insomnia, anti-proliferative, anti-anxiety & anti-oxidant
Also Found In:
lilac, tea tree, nutmeg, pine trees, apples, cumin & cannabis

Endocannabinoid System
The Endocannabinoid System Explained

This is an overview of how cannabis affects the body. Your body consists of various systems, including a crucial internal regulator system known as the endocannabinoid system. Cannabis can interact with this system by introducing cannabinoids such as THC and CBD, which bind to receptors (called CB1 & CB2 which awesomely already exist in the human body) in our cells and generate a range of therapeutic effects.

The endocannabinoid system helps to regulate key functions, such as the immune and nervous systems, through a complex network of molecules and receptors. This widespread receptor system is believed to be the largest in the body, playing a crucial role in maintaining many fundamental physiological processes, including pain sensation, immunity, inflammation, blood pressure, memory, and appetite, among others. Scientists speculate that the endocannabinoid system originated in early animals more than 600 million years ago.

The Human Endocannabinoid System helps to regulate your bodily function. Take a look at what each receptor does for your body.

CB1 Receptors Target:
Motor Activity
Thinking
Motor Coordination
Appetite
Short-Term Memory
Pain Perception
Immune Cells

CB2 Receptors Target:
Gut
Kidneys
Pancreas
Adipose Tissue
Skeletal Muscle
Bone
Eye
Tumors
Reproductive System
Respiratory Tract
Immune System
Skin
Central Nervous System
Cardiovascular System
Liver

Methods of Administration

In this segment you'll learn about the different routes in which you can receive cannabis in the body as well as the duration and peak times for each. In our book, you'll mainly use sublingual and edible. However, we encourage you to explore the other methods below as you read along and create our various recipes. We'll spark one up with ya - pun intended :)

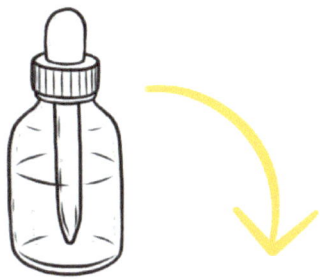

SUBLINGUAL ADMINISTRATION

Sublingual forms are administered under the tongue and may be faster acting as the medicine is absorbed into the blood through the mucosal membrane in the mouth.

Peak effect: 15 minutes
Duration: 6 - 8 hours

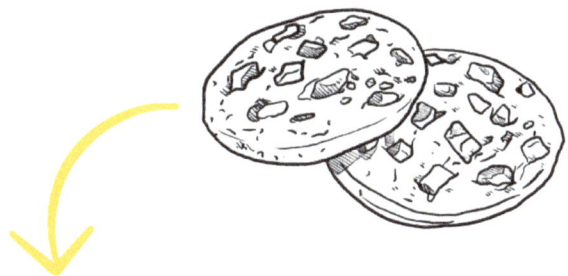

EDIBLE ADMINISTRATION

Edibles need to be digested in order for your body to process them. More precisely, they need to reach the small intestine and the liver. As soon as they arrive there, the fats in the edibles are broken down and finally passed into the bloodstream to supply th body with nutrients, cannabinoids and other substances.

Peak effect: 1 - 2 hours
Duration: 4 - 6 hours

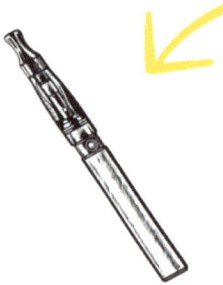

VAPORIZING ADMINISTRATION
Inhalation through vaporization is the fastest-acting method of administration. When inhaled, the active ingredients of the product pass directly into the bloodstream from the lungs.
Peak effect: 15 - 30 minutes
Duration: 2 - 3 hours

TOPICAL ADMINISTRATION
Topical forms are typically used as creams, balms, ointments, lotions, oils or salves to manage any discomfort, delivering active ingredients to the bloodstream through the skin.
Peak effect: 0 - 30 minutes
Duration: 1 - 4 hours

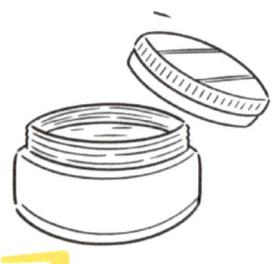

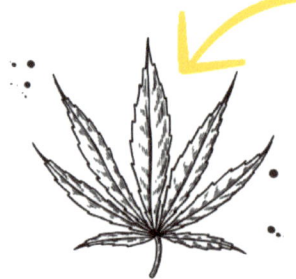

SMOKEABLE ADMINISTRATION
When the cannabis flower is smoked, THC, CBD and other phyto-cannabinoids, as well as terpenes, are vaporized by the heat of combustion and inhaled. This provides the whole plant benefit, known as the "entourage effect." Inhaled active ingredients are quickly passed from the lungs into the bloodstream.
Peak effect: 15 - 30 minutes
Duration: 2 - 3 hours

ORAL ADMINISTRATION
Oral administration is one of the strongest delivery methods out there. Unlike inhaled cannabis, ingested cannabis is metabolized b the liver. This means that more THC is converted into usable forms by the body.
Peak effect: 2 - 6 hours
Duration: 4 - 12 hours

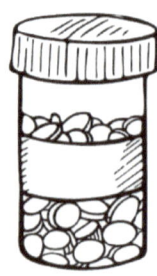

Infusion Methods

36	Concentrates & Flower
37	Decarboxylation
38	Infused Agave, Honey & Maple Syrup
39	Infused Butter
40	Infused Compound Butter
41	Infused Cooking Oil
42	Infused Tinctures
43	Dosage Calculation

There are many wonderful ways to infuse your lifestyle with cannabis. This chapter will teach you how we do it.

Be sure to especially take note of the "Dosage Calculation" chapter. The recipes in our book give you the option to choose your infusion method.

Some recipes will allow for multiple infusion options to choose from. Always pay attention to the amounts your infusin with to never over do it. Trust, that won't be a pleasant experience.

Concentrates & Flower

There are multiple ways to skin a cow or do a math problem so why expect anything different from cannabis? Since cannabis became widely known for its healing properties, more and more infusion and extraction methods have become more widely sought after.

Dosing with cannabis can be tricky for beginners and finicky for some. To us, the key to finding the right dosage meant for you, is to **start low and slow**. You can always up your dosage once you've got a better handle on where you like to be with your cannabis infused lifestyle.

Always follow label instructions for serving suggestions. **Do not** let anyone pressure you into taking more than you know you can handle. Just because it tastes great does not mean eat the entire thing.

The fastest way to consume cannabis is to inhale it. However, studies shows how in the long run this method is not always best. This method burns most of the cannabis away before you can consume it and the effects usually do not last very long.

Flower/Kief
You can decarboxylate your cannabis buds to activate it, grind it up and add it to anything. Make your very own canna-flour using this method.

Distillate or Isolate
This infusion methods is the easiest way to dose and infuse your favorite foods.

Wax/Crumble
A little goes a long way with this one. We recommend this method for experienced cannabis users.

Oil/Butter Infusions
This is where your now decarboxylated bud gets infused into your favorite oil and/or butter. There are multiple ways to do this at home right in your kitchen.

RSO/Tincture
Again, a little goes a long way with this one too. We use this method for liquids like tea, soup or juices. These two methods are user friendly for everyone. Just follow the dosage instructions on the label.

Decarboxylation

To begin, you are going to need to decarboxylate your cannabis flower. It is the similar process as when you light yo joint, blunt or bowl to smoke. This process activates the cannabinoids in the cannabis, making them bioavailable. (Example: THCA becomes THC once it's undergone this process)

To do this, you can either purchase a machine that will do it f you or do it in your oven at home. We use the Ardent FX Decarboxylating Machine. It's about $300 and well worth the price. Especially if you don't feel comfortable attempting to d this in your oven on your own

Trust the Process!

Low & slow is the key for doing this process without proper machinery. There are plenty of YouTube videos/blogs on ho to decarboxylate your your flower so we won't get into fine detail here.

Once this step has been done, proceed to infuse using the Ardent FX Machine or on your stove top pot with simmering water & place a mason jar with lid on it for about two hours.

Once finished, strain into a reliable container & keep straine flowers as well. We like to cook our meals with it every now a then. After all, you can't possibly get everything out by hand. You'll thank us later!

{FAIR WARNING: THE DECARB PROCESS BEING DONE IN YO OVEN AT HOME WILL NOT GIVE THE SAME ACCURATE RESULTS SO WE RECOMMEND YOU INVEST IN A MACHINE THAT WILL DO IT FOR YOU}

Infused Honey, Agave & Maple Syrup

> Honey and maple syrup are staples in our household. We pretty much use them on everything. Agave, of course, is a more ethically sourced option if you're concerned about the Bee's or want to make an outstanding margarita. Naturally, honey, agave, and maple syrup also make great mediums to infuse into your recipes—not to mention the unique health benefits each one offers.
>
> **PRO TIP:** Go a step further by adding dried lavender leaves or any other dried herb of your choice to brighten the flavor.

Ingredients & Equipment:

- 4 grams Decarboxylated Cannabis (ex. whole buds, shake, etc.)
- 8 ounces Honey, Agave or Maple Syrup

- Saucepan or double boiler
- Heat-resistant bowl
- Fine-mesh strainer or cheesecloth
- Spatula
- Glass container with lid

OR Ardent or Levo Infusion Machine (optional)

Directions:

1. **Infuse the honey.** In a double boiler or a heat-resistant bowl placed over a saucepan with simmering water, combine the honey and decarboxylated cannabis. Stir to mix them together.
2. **Heat gently.** Maintain a low heat and let the mixture simmer for about 2 hours, stirring occasionally. This allows the cannabinoids to infuse into the honey. Ensure the heat is low to avoid scorching the honey or cannabis.
3. **Strain the honey.** Set a fine-mesh strainer or cheesecloth over a heat-resistant bowl. Pour the infused honey through the strainer to separate the plant material from the liquid. Press down gently on the cannabis to extract any remaining honey.
4. **Cool and store.** Allow the infused honey to cool to room temperature. Then, transfer it to an airtight container for storage. Store it in a cool, dark place, such as a pantry or refrigerator.

***Exchange "honey" in the directions interchangeably if you're using agave or maple syrup instead.

Infused Butter

> Butter is, by far, the most popular way to infuse your recipes with cannabis, second only to oil. When it comes to choosing your butter, we prefer unsalted, which gives us more control over the flavor outcome, as well as ensuring a good quality product. Of course, you can use store-branded butter, or you can even go as far as making butter from scratch first. You might even opt for an already flavored butter. No matter what you choose, here's how we like to infuse it.

Ingredients & Equipment:

- 16 grams Decarboxylated Cannabis (ex. whole buds, shake, etc.)
- 1 pound Unsalted Butter
- Freshly Ground Black Pepper & Salt (or seasonings of your choice)

- Saucepan or double boiler
- Heat-resistant bowl
- Fine-mesh strainer or cheesecloth
- Spatula
- Glass container with lid or preferably silicone molds for storage which makes infusing easier

OR Ardent or Levo Infusion Machine (optional)

Directions:

1. **Melt the butter.** In a saucepan or double boiler, melt the unsalted butter over low heat. Stir occasionally to ensure even melting and prevent burning.
2. **Add the decarboxylated cannabis.** Once the butter has melted, add the decarboxylated cannabis to the saucepan. Stir to combine, ensuring all the cannabis is coated with butter.
3. **Infuse the butter.** Simmer the mixture on low heat for 2-3 hours, stirring occasionally. This allows the cannabinoids to infuse into the butter. Ensure the heat is low to avoid scorching the butter or cannabis.
4. **Strain the butter.** Set a fine-mesh strainer or cheesecloth over a heat-resistant bowl. Pour the infused butter through the strainer to separate the plant material from the liquid. Press down gently on the cannabis to extract any remaining butter.
5. **Storage.** Pour strained butter into preferred storage vessel.
6. **Cool and solidify.** Allow the infused butter to cool to room temperature. Then, transfer it to the refrigerator to solidify. This process usually takes a few hours, depending on the amount of butter.
7. **Store the infused butter.** Once the butter has solidified, transfer it to an airtight container for storage. Keep it in the refrigerator or freezer, where it can last for several weeks or even months.

Infused Compound Butter

Elevate your butter by transforming it into compound butter. While you can certainly buy pre-flavored butter from the store, rest assure that this homemade variation surpasses it.

Ingredients & Equipment:
- Infused Butter, slightly chilled (from previous page)
- Freshly Ground Black Pepper & Salt (or seasonings of your choice)
- Roasted Garlic or Freshly Crushed Garlic
- Fresh Herbs of your choice

- Food Processor

OR mixing bowl with spatula

OR Stand mixer fitted with a paddle
- Cutting board & Knife
- Glass container with lid or preferably silicone molds for storage which makes infusing easier

Directions:
1. **Soften the butter.** Take the desired amount of unsalted butter out of the refrigerator and let it sit at room temperature until it softens. It should be soft enough to easily mix but not melted.
2. **Prepare the flavorings.** Decide on the flavors you want to add to your compound butter. This can include herbs, spices, garlic, citrus zest, or other ingredients. Finely chop or mince the flavorings so that they incorporate evenly into the butter.

By Hand:
- Combine butter and flavorings: In a mixing bowl, add the softened butter and the prepared flavorings. Use a spoon or spatula to thoroughly mix the butter and flavorings together until well combined.

Using a Stand Mixer:
- Cream the butter: Place the softened butter in the mixing bowl of a stand mixer fitted with the paddle attachment. Beat the butter on medium speed until it becomes smooth and creamy.
- Add the flavorings: Reduce the mixer speed to low, and gradually add the prepared flavorings to the creamed butter. Allow the mixer to run until the flavorings are evenly distributed throughout the butter.

Using a Food Processor:
- Add butter and flavorings: Place the softened butter and the prepared flavorings into the bowl of a food processor.
- Process until combined: Pulse the food processor in short bursts until the butter and flavorings are thoroughly mixed and form a cohesive mixture. Scrape down the sides of the bowl as needed.

Storage. No matter the method chosen, aim to use silicone molds for storage which makes infusing easier. Simply evenly portion your butter using a spatula.

Infused Cooking Oil

> Infused cooking oil is perfect if you prefer not to use butter or have dietary restrictions. When choosing your oil, it's best to select a high-quality oil that is also nutritious. We typically prefer to infuse with either coconut oil, grapeseed oil, or extra virgin olive oil. Grapeseed oil contains high levels of Vitamin E, has antioxidant properties, and a high smoke point, which makes it suitable for high-temperature cooking. Our two favorites among the three mentioned are grapeseed and extra virgin olive oil.
>
> **PRO TIP:** Add roasted garlic or other herbs like oregano to create a savory flavor. This is a great way to infuse all of your meals.

Ingredients & Equipment:

- 12 grams Decarboxylated Cannabis (ex. whole buds, shake, etc.)
- 12 ounces Grapeseed or Extra Virgin Olive Oil

- Glass jar with a tight-fitting lid
- Fine-mesh strainer or cheesecloth
- Funnel
- Oil dispensing bottle glass for storage (makes infusing easier)

OR Ardent or Levo Infusion Machine (optional)

Directions:

1. **Grind your cannabis.** This will help infuse the oil more effectively.
2. **Place your cannabis flower in a jar.** Transfer to a glass jar with a tight-fitting lid. Make sure the jar is clean and dry.
3. **Add oil.** Pour the oil over the your cannabis flower, ensuring that it covers the herb completely.
4. **Seal the jar.** Securely close the jar with the lid and give it a gentle shake to combine the ingredients.
5. **Infuse the oil.** Heat the jar in a double boiler on low heat for 2 hours. This is achieved by filling a small to medium sauce pot halfway with water and placing jar inside. Ensure the water covers the level of the mixture inside throughout the infusion process.
6. **Strain the oil.** After the infusion period, strain the oil to remove the cannabis matter. Line a fine-mesh strainer or cheesecloth over a funnel and place it over a clean glass jar or bowl. Pour the infused oil through the strainer, allowing it to filter out the herb particles. Press down gently on the cannabis matter to extract any remaining liquid. (PRO TIP: Save pressed cannabis matter for compound butter)
7. **Bottle and store.** Use a funnel to transfer the strained oil into a oil dispensing bottle for storage. Label the bottle with the date and contents.
8. **Storage.** Store the cannabis infused oil in a cool, dark place. When stored properly, it can last for several months. However, it's advisable to check for any signs of spoilage before use.

Infused Tincture

> An infused tincture is the most versatile and easiest to use of all the infusion methods mentioned previously. You can discreetly travel with it and use it for a variety of infusions, such as coffee, tea, mocktails, soup, salad, etc. You can even dose with this method by taking the dropper directly under your tongue.
>
> PRO TIP: To add a savory flavor to your meals, consider infusing your tincture with roasted garlic or other herbs like oregano.

Ingredients & Equipment:

- 3 grams Decarboxylated Cannabis (ex. whole buds, shake, etc.)
- 1 ounce MCT Oil (Medium Chain Triglycerides)

- Glass jar with a tight-fitting lid
- Fine-mesh strainer or cheesecloth
- Funnel
- 30ml Amber glass dropper bottles for storage

OR Ardent or Levo Infusion Machine (optional)

Directions:

1. **Grind your cannabis.** This will help infuse the oil more effectively.
2. **Place your cannabis flower in a jar.** Transfer to a glass jar with a tight-fitting lid. Make sure the jar is clean and dry.
3. **Add MCT oil.** Pour the MCT oil over the your cannabis flower, ensuring that it covers the herb completely.
4. **Seal the jar.** Securely close the jar with the lid and give it a gentle shake to combine the ingredients.
5. **Infuse the tincture.** Heat the jar in a double boiler on low heat for 2 hours. This is achieved by filling a small to medium sauce pot halfway with water and placing jar inside. Ensure the water covers the level of the mixture inside throughout the infusion process.
6. **Strain the tincture.** After the infusion period, strain the tincture to remove the cannabis matter. Line a fine-mesh strainer or cheesecloth over a funnel and place it over a clean glass jar or bowl. Pour the infused oil through the strainer, allowing it to filter out the herb particles. Press down gently on the cannabis matter to extract any remaining liquid. (PRO TIP: Save pressed cannabis matter for compound butter)
7. **Bottle and store.** Use a funnel to transfer the strained tincture into amber glass bottles for storage. Amber glass helps protect the tincture from light degradation. Label the bottle with the date and contents.
8. **Storage.** Store the cannabis infused MCT oil in a cool, dark place. When stored properly, it can last for several months. However, it's advisable to check for any signs of spoilage before use.

Dosage Calculation

> Bookmark this page for future reference and guidance on dosing with our ratios. Or adjust the ratio for the dosage as you see fit. For example, you want double potency, simply double the amount of cannabis used in the same amount of butter, oil, honey, etc. called for in the recipe. Important tip: please be mindful that these are genaral approximations. If you have access to cannabis with acurate milligrams, adjust our ratios to to fit your needs.

Honey, Agave or Maple Syrup

Our recipe for these mediums use a 1:2 ratio

Total amount = approximately 400 milligrams
1 ounce = approximately 50 milligrams
1 tablespoon = approximately 25 milligrams
1 teaspoon = approximately 8 milligrams

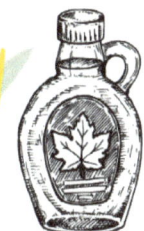

Butter

Our recipe for this medium uses a 1:1 ratio

Total amount = approximately 1,600 milligrams
1/4 cup = approximately 200 milligrams
1 ounce = approximately 100 milligrams
1 tablespoon = approximately 50 milligrams

Cooking Oil

Our recipe for this medium uses a 1:1 ratio

Total amount = approximately 1,200 milligrams
1 ounce = approximately 100 milligrams
1 tablespoon = approximately 50 milligrams
1 teaspoon = approximately 16 milligrams

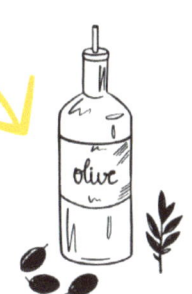

Tincture

Our recipe for this medium uses a 3:1 ratio
The 1 ounce dropper bottle contains appx. 30 full droppers

Total amount = approximately 300 milligrams
1 tablespoon = approximately 150 milligrams
1 full dropper = approximately 10 milligrams
1/2 dropper = approximately 5 milligrams

Breads & Dough

45	Focaccia Bread
46	Garlic Bread
47	Pasta Dough
48	Pancakes or Waffles
49	Pizza Dough
50	Sweet Dinner Rolls

This chapter is a great introduction to bread making. If you own a bread maker-good for you-but we will be using our stand KitchenAid mixer (or whatever stand mixer you have).

However, if you do not own one of these, do not fret, these recipes are so simple that they can also be made by hand with a spoon and a bowl.

Focaccia Bread

This is hands down one of our favorite breads to make. It's not only absolutely delicious, but also highly versatile for alternative recipe variations. You can combine the ingredients in your stand mixer or easily mix by hand.

Prep Time: 75 Minutes
Bake Time: 20 Minutes
Yield: 8

Infusion Options:
Cannabis Honey or Cannabis Oil

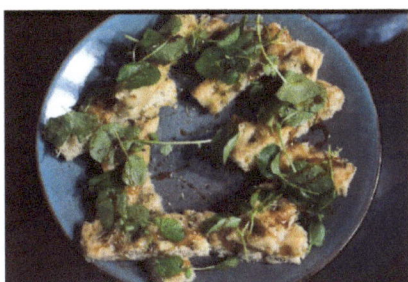

Ingredients:

- 9.3 ounces Warm Water (About 110°F)
- 2 teaspoons Pure Honey
- 1 (0.25 ounce) Package Active-Dry Yeast
- 438 grams Unbleached All-Purpose Flour
- 2 ounces Extra Virgin Olive Oil, Plus More For Drizzling
- 2 teaspoons Sea Salt
- 2 sprigs Fresh Rosemary

Directions:

1. **Proof the yeast**. Add the warm water, which you can measure with your thermometer. Stir in the honey and the yeast. Let this mixture develop for 5 to 10 minutes.
2. **Knead the dough.** Mix on low speed or by hand and gradually add flour, olive oil and salt. Increase speed to medium-low, and continue mixing the dough for 5 minutes. (If the dough is too sticky and isn't pulling away from the sides of the bowl or forming by hand, add in an extra 30 grams of flour while it is mixing.)
3. **First dough rise.** Once your dough has formed a smooth surface, form into a ball, place in a greased bowl, cover it with a damp towel and let the dough rise for 45-60 minutes, or until it has nearly doubled in size.
4. **Second dough rise.** Turn the dough onto a floured surface, and roll it out into a large circle or rectangle until that the dough is about 1/2-inch thick*. Cover the dough again with the damp towel, and let the dough continue to rise for another 20 minutes.
5. **Prepare the dough.** Preheat oven to 400°F. Transfer the dough to a large parchment-covered baking sheet. Use your fingers to poke deep dents all over the surface of the dough. Drizzle a tablespoon or two of olive oil evenly all over the top of the dough, and sprinkle evenly with the fresh rosemary and sea salt.
6. **Bake.** Bake for 20 minutes, or until the dough is slightly golden and cooked through.
7. **Serve.** Remove from the oven, and drizzle with a little more olive oil if desired. Slice, and serve warm.

Variations: Add or swap in freshly diced garlic, baby tomatoes, and/or any other fresh herbs. Use either Cannabis Honey or Cannabis Oil to infuse this recipe.

Garlic Bread

This recipe is a classic using a Basic Lean Dough recipe. Enjoy this recipe all on its own, pair with an awesome seafood dip, or with your favorite pasta or soup recipe. Combine in your stand mixer or mix by hand.

Prep Time: 55 Minutes
Bake Time: 30 Minutes
Yield: 12 to 16

Infusion Options:
Cannabis Butter or Cannabis Oil

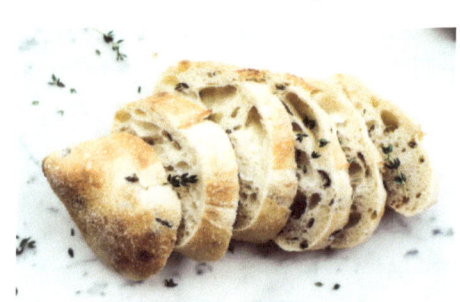

Ingredients:

For the bread:
- 7 ounces Warm Water (About 110°F)
- 1 tablespoon Active Dry Yeast
- 330 grams Unbleached Bread Flour
- 1 teaspoon Sea Salt

For the topping:
- 3 cloves Fresh Garlic
- 2 tablespoons Olive Oil
- 2 sticks Unsalted Butter
- 2 tablespoons Fresh Parsley, Minced

Directions:

1. **For the bread.** Combine water, yeast, flour and salt in stand mixer or by hand in a bowl.
2. **Knead the dough.** Mix on low speed or by hand about 4 minutes. Turn out the dough onto a floured surface and knead the dough for another 5 minutes.(If the dough is too sticky and isn't pulling away from the sides of the bowl or forming by hand, add in an extra 30 grams of flour while it is mixing.)
3. **Let dough rise.** Once your dough has formed a smooth surface, form into a ball, place in a flour dusted bowl, cover it with a damp towel and let the dough rise for 45-60 minutes, or until it has nearly doubled in size.
4. **Divide the dough and rest.** Turn the dough onto a floured surface, and divide into smaller equal pieces or leave it whole. Pre-shape the dough into a round oval. Rest the dough for another 20 to 30 minutes.
5. **Prepare the dough.** Preheat oven to 400°F. Shape dough into final rounded log and transfer the dough to a large parchment-covered baking sheet. Use a sharp blade to lightly slice seams on just the surface of the dough diagonally (about 3 to 4).
6. **Bake.** Bake for 20 to 25 minutes, or until the dough is slightly golden and cooked through. Once cooled, slice into 1" rounds and place back on baking sheet.
7. **For the topping.** Combine oil, butter and garlic into a small blender to make a garlic paste. Spread this mix on top of each round and top evenly with the minced parsley.
8. **Bake again and serve.** Finish with fresh black pepper and a pinch of salt.

Variations: Top with parmesan cheese (vegan or not) prior to baking the second time. Use either cannabis oil or cannabis butter to infuse this recipe. How To Infuse: Replace the butter or oil in this recipe with infused butter or oil.

Pasta Dough

Making pasta dough from scratch might seem overwhelming, but we promise you, it's incredibly easy and quick. Fresh pasta is unparalleled compared to store-bought varieties. You can easily combine these ingredients in a bowl, stand mixer or on a clean surface by hand.

Prep Time: 55 Minutes
Yield: 4 Servings

Infusion Options:
Cannabis Oil or
Decarboxylated Flower/Kief

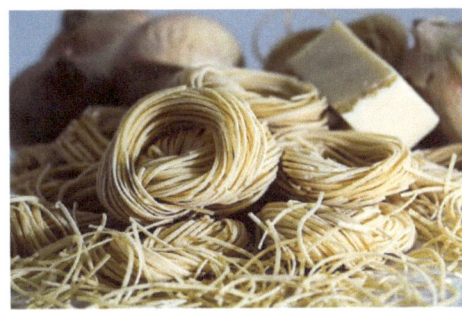

Ingredients:

- 6 ounces Water, (you might need a little more)
- 1 tablespoon Extra Virgin Olive Oil
- 426 grams Unbleached All-Purpose Flour
- 1 teaspoon Sea Salt

Directions:

1. **Scale.** Gather and combine all of your ingredients together until it forms a rough dough.
2. **A lot of kneading.** You can begin mixing this in your stand mixer but honestly, this recipe is so easy that doing this by hand works perfectly fine. You'll want to keep kneading until the dough forms a smooth ball.
3. **Rest.** The dough needs to rest for a minimum of 30 minutes at room temperature or overnight in the refrigerator. Wrap in plastic and make sure its completely covered.
4. **Divide.** Portion into two pieces and keep one half covered in plastic wrap on the counter. Using your rolling pin roll out the dough until its thin enough to go into your pasta attachment. If you don't have a pasta attachment, keep on rolling until it is thin enough to your liking.
5. **Shaping.** Have fun with this part. There's so many possibilities here. You can make noodles to stuffed raviolis and so many other varieties in between.
6. **Dry out or cook.** Fresh pasta does not take as long to boil as store bought pasta. Boil for about 2 minutes and drain. If you're not cooking the pasta tonight, dry out on a pasta drying rack or on a sheet tray with parchment paper.

Variations: Add in ground dried or fresh herbs to your all-purpose flour. To infuse incorporate your decarboxylated flower or kief into the flour or if you're using tincture mix it in with the wet ingredients.

Pancakes or Waffles

If you like to start your morning off elevated, you'll love these easy to make fluffy pancakes. Pro tip: DO NOT use old baking powder.

Prep Time: 25 Minutes
Cook Time: 30 Minutes
Yield: 4 - 6 Medium Pancakes

Infusion Options:
Cannabis Tincture or
Decarboxylated Flower/Kief

Ingredients:

- 130 grams Unbleached All-Purpose Flour
- 2 tablespoons Cane Sugar or Light Brown Sugar
- 1/2 tablespoon Baking Powder
- ½ teaspoon Salt
- 7 ounces Oat Milk
- 1/2 tablespoon Apple Cider Vinegar
- 1 teaspoon Pure Vanilla Extract
- Ground Cinnamon, Optional
- Maple Syrup, To Serve

Bump up your infusion by also using infused maple syrup and/or infused cannabis butter once your pancakes or waffles are ready to eat.

Directions:

1. **In a medium bowl**, add the flour, sugar, baking powder, and salt, and stir to combine.
2. **In a medium bowl** or liquid measuring cup, add oat milk, apple cider vinegar, and vanilla, and stir to combine. Let this liquid mixture rest for 3 minutes before addinf to dry ingredients. This is your "buttermilk". (If you woukd like to just use buttermilk, omit the apple cider vinegar.
3. **Pour the liquid** mixture into the dry mixture and stir. DO NOT OVERMIX.
4. **Let batter rest** for 5 minutes. Batter should look lumpy and thick not runny and thin.
5. **Pour** about ½ cup (65 grams) of batter onto a nonstick pan or griddle over medium heat.
6. **When** the top begins to bubble, flip the pancake and cook until golden.
7. **For waffles,** heat a waffle maker, spray with nonstick oil, pour batter in and cook thoroughly until is ready to your liking.
8. **Serve warm** with maple syrup.

Variations: Add your favorite toppings like strawberries, blueberries, chocolate chips, banana or oats. To infuse, add in ground dried or fresh herbs to your all-purpose flour. To infuse incorporate your decarboxylated flower or kief into the flour or if you're using tincture mix it in with the wet ingredients.

Pizza Dough

Of course you can just order a pizza and have it delivered right to your door but there's so much satisfaction in making it yourself-especially when it's both infused and easy to make.

Prep Time: 25 Minutes
Cook Time: 30 Minutes
Yield: 2 Medium or 1 Large

Infusion Options:
Cannabis Oil or
Decarboxylated Flower/Kief

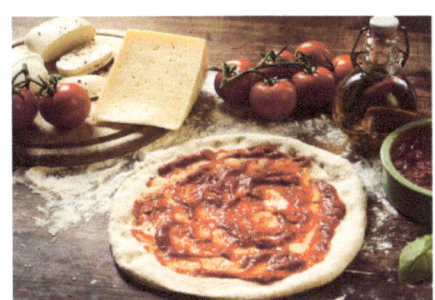

Ingredients:

- 2 ¼ cups All-Purpose Flour
- 1 teaspoon Sugar
- 1 teaspoon Salt
- 2 ¼ teaspoons Active Dry Yeast
- ¾ cup Warm Water (around 110°F/43°C)
- 2 tablespoons Olive Oil

Directions:

1. Mix 2 ¼ cups flour, 1 tsp sugar, and 1 tsp salt in a bowl.
2. In a small bowl, dissolve 2 ¼ tsp yeast in ¾ cup warm water. Let it sit for 5 minutes until foamy.
3. Add the yeast mixture and 2 tbsp olive oil to the dry ingredients. Stir until combined.
4. Knead the dough on a lightly floured surface for 5-7 minutes until smooth and elastic.
5. Shape the dough into a ball and place it in a greased bowl. Cover and let it rise for 1 hour or until doubled in size.
6. Punch down the dough to remove air bubbles.
7. Divide the dough into 2 portions for medium pizzas or leave as one portion for a large pizza.
8. Roll out each portion on a floured surface to the desired thickness.
9. Transfer the dough to a pizza stone, baking sheet, or peel lined with parchment paper.
10. Add your favorite toppings. Bake at 475°F (245°C) for 12-15 minutes or until golden and bubbly.
11. Let it cool for a few minutes, then slice and enjoy!

Feel free to customize the recipe by adding your preferred herbs or spices to the dough. Enjoy your homemade pizza. Use either cannabis oi or decarboxylated flower/kief to infuse this recipe.

Sweet Dinner Rolls

This recipe is traditionally a braided bread and is one of the most popular and frequently consumed breads in Guyanese cuisine originally named "Plait Bread". It is usually made for stew during the holidays but I make this bread throughout the year in so many ways.

Bake Time: 30 Minutes
Yield: 4 Servings

Infusion Option:
Cannabis Butter

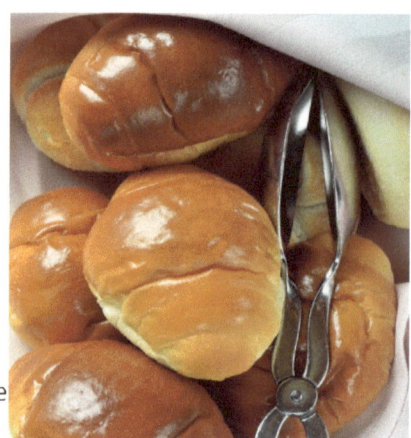

Ingredients:

- 410 grams Unbleached All-Purpose Flour
- 10 ounces Warm Water
- 75 grams Dark Brown Sugar
- 1 tablespoon Dry Active Yeast
- 1/2 teaspoon Salt
- 1/2 stick Unsalted Butter, Room Temperature

Extra Butter, To Top & Serve.

Directions:

1. **Scale.** Gather and combine all of your ingredients together until it forms a rough dough.
2. **You can begin mixing** this in your stand mixer but honestly, this recipe is so easy that doing this by hand works perfectly fine. You'll want to keep kneading until the dough forms a smooth ball being careful not to over-knead.
3. **Let dough rise.** Once your dough has formed a smooth surface, form into a ball, place in a flour dusted bowl, cover it with a damp towel and let the dough rise for 45-60 minutes, or until it has nearly doubled in size.
4. **If you have a kitchen scale,** weigh the total dough and divide the dough evenly. If you don't have one, simply divide the dough into 3-4 inch rolls. Once there all shaped, place them on a baking tray and let these rise again until doubled in size. During this time, make sure to preheat your oven to 350 degrees Fahrenheit.
5. **You can brush more butter** on before you bake. The rolls should take anywhere between 25 to 30 minutes. Once theyre out of the oven, immediately brush more butter on the surface. For added sugary crunch, add a dusting of cane sugar on top of the butter.
6. **Serve immediately** or store in an air tight bread bag and/or container.

How To Infuse: You can use cannabis butter or cannabis honey. Use cannabis butter within this recipe or use the cannabis honey after th rolls are baked as a topping.

Stocks & Sauces

52	No Waste Vegetable Stock
53	Bone Broth
54	Brown Butter Alfredo Sauce
55	Garlic Roasted Pizza Sauce
56	Presto Pesto Sauce
57	Oven Roasted Tomato Sauce

Stocks are where true recipes are born. Stocks add a wonderful essence to what you are cooking. It gives more flavor, more dept and more life without overpowering anything else. Think of it this way, why add water when you can add broth?

On the other hand, the sauce is what brings it all together. Sauces have the ability to move the flavor you want across the entire dish or be explosion of flavor you were looking for on the side.

No Waste Vegetable Stock

This page is essential to every recipe you will make in this book and more. Nothing is waste or trash. Here you will see the beauty in saving edible scraps.

Prep Time: 30 Minutes Over 1 Week Period
Cook Time: At Least 12 Hours

Infusion Options:
Cannabis Tincture or Cooking Oil
or Cannabis Butter
or Decarboxylated Flower/Kief

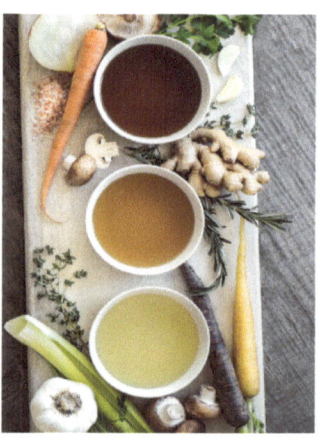

Ingredients Are Variable(s):

Save every and all:

garlic scraps/skin, onion scraps/skin, tomato scraps, carrot scraps, veggie scraps, cucumber scraps, fresh herb stalks, ginger skin peels, corn peel/stalks, orange peels, lemon peel, almost bad salad leaves, spinach, kale, lettuce, arugula, fruit scraps/peels, assorted nuts, etc.

Directions:

1. **In a medium to large stock pot**, add all of your saved vegetable scraps/skin/peel along with filtered water, kosher salt and black pepper.
2. **Boil this mixture**, stir ocassionally, until the mixture reduces by half.
3. **Add more water**, as if filling back up again and reduce further than halfway this time.
4. **Strain out scraps** and add salt & fresh cracked black pepper to taste.
5. **Let broth cool** or serve right away for homemade vegetable broth with ramen. Save this broth recipe for other everyday favorites like making rice, pasta, quinoa, soup, or any recipe that calls for water.

How To Infuse: Add your favorite dose of tincture, infused cooking oil/butter or activated ground flower/kief for your own portion or enough to serve the group. Our recommended single dose is any where between 5mg to 25mg per person per dose.

Bone Broth

The beauty of this broth is the level of flavor that no vegetable broth could ever achieve. The secret is in the bone marrow that is extracted and infused into the broth along with the animal fat leaving a beautiful layer of delicious gelatin. No matter what bone or crustacean shell you have, YOU'LL WANT TO SAVE IT FOR THIS!

Prep Time: 30 Minutes Over 1 Week Period
Cook Time: At Least 12 Hours

Infusion Options:
Cannabis Tincture or Cooking Oil
or Cannabis Butter
or Decarboxylated Flower/Kief

Ingredients Are Variable(s):

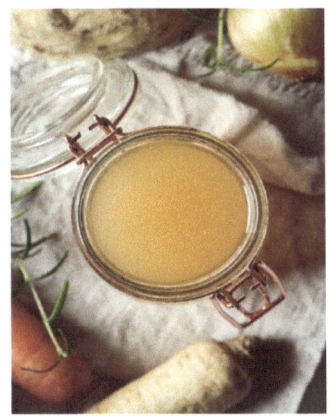

Save every and all:

garlic scraps/skin, onion scraps/skin, tomato scraps, carrot scraps, veggie scraps, cucumber scraps, fresh herb stalks, ginger skin peels, corn peel/stalks, orange peels, lemon peel, almost bad salad leaves, spinach, kale, lettuce, arugula, fruit scraps/peels, assorted nuts, etc.

Plus your favorite collection of animal fat(s) like from bacon, bones from chicken/turkey, t-bone from the steak or bone-in from a ribeye, any and all bone scraps from deboning a fish or shells from crustaceans, etc.

Directions:

1. **In a medium to large stock pot**, add all of your saved vegetable scraps/skin/peel and animal scraps along with filtered water, kosher salt and black pepper. Feel free to add in additional flavor in like Old Bay or broth seasoning cubes.
2. **Boil this mixture**, stirring ocassionally, until the mixture reuces by half.
3. **Add more water**, as if filling back up again and reduce further than halfway this time.
4. **Add salt &** fresh cracked black pepper to taste.
5. **Let broth cool** or serve right away for homemade bone broth with ramen. Save this broth recipe for other everyday favorites like making, rice, pasta, quinoa, soup, or any recipe that calls for water.

How To Infuse: Add your favorite dose of tincture, infused cooking oil/butter or activated ground flower/kief for your own portion or enough to serve the group. Our recommended single dose is any where between 10mg to 25mg per person.

Brown Butter Alfredo Sauce

This recipe is home for us. It is the very first infused sauce we've ever created together. The browning of the butter is the most lucritive part of this recipe so don't skip it and please don't burn it..

Prep Time: 30 Minutes
Oven Time: 10 Minutes

Infusion Options:
Cannabis Tincture or Cannabis Butter

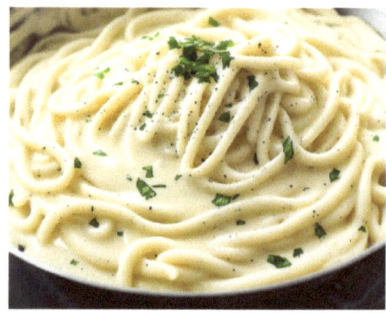

Ingredients:

- 1 stick Unsalted Butter, Browned
- 1 quart Heavy Cream
- 1/2 cups of pasta water
- 2 sprigs of Fresh Oregano
- 1 sprig of Fresh Rosemary
- 1 1/2 teaspoon Dried, Basil
- 1/2 each Small White Onion, Diced
- 1 each Shallot, Diced
- 2 teaspoons Smoked Paprika
- 1/2 cup White Chardonnay Wine
- 1 cup Cheese, Shredded

Salt & Fresh Cracked Black Pepper T.T.

Directions:

1. **In a small sauce pot**, add your stick of butter and simmer on medium heat, stirring occasionally. You will know when your butter is ready by color, smell and taste. The color should be golden brown, it should smell roasted/nutty and when cooled, it should taste toasty and nutty. Make sure to strain brown butter with a fine mesh and/or cheesecloth to ensure impurities are removed.
2. **To a medium to large sauce pot**, add in your browned butter, diced shallots and diced white onion. While this simmers, add in your smoked paprika and dried basil.
3. **Next,** use kitchen twine to make a bouquet garnet to wrap your fresh oregano and fresh rosemary in a cheesecloth bundle. This technique is used for when you want the flavor and not the particles in your sauce.
4. **Add in your heavy cream,** oregano/rosemary herb bundle and let this mixture reduce halfway. Then add in your wine and cheese(s) and let this reduce one more time. Remove bouquet garnet and blend sauce together with emulsion blender.
5. **Serve with** cooked pasta and chicken and/or mushrooms right away or store in an air tight container in the fridge or freezer. Please note that once chilled, the sauce will be a thicker paste consistency. Reheat this sauce in a sauce pan on low heat until creamy and saucy.

How To Infuse: You will either add cannabis into your brown butter or infuse your already browned butter with cannabis. **Vegan Variation:** Sub butter and cheese for vegan butter and cheese. Also sub the heavy cream for full-fat coconut cream. To properly make vegan browned butter, you'll need to repeat step one plus add in pecans. Pecans give the nutty flavor component that non-vegan butter creates on its own.

Garlic Roasted Pizza Sauce

Yes there's pizza sauce but there's our pizza sauce! Your canned tomato recipe will never measure up to this. It can try but it won't!

Prep Time: 10 Minutes
Cook Time: 2 Hours
Yield: Appx. 2 Cups

Infusion Options:
Cannabis Tincture or Cannabis Oil or Cannabis Honey

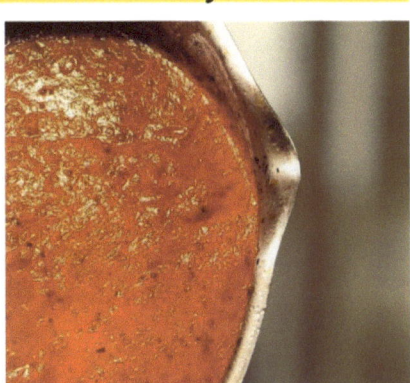

Ingredients:

- 8 each Tomatoes On The Vine, Uncut
- 3 each Fresh Garlic Cloves, Uncut
- 1/4 cup Grapeseed Oil
- 1/4 cup Dried Basil and Dried Oregano
- 1 cup Kale Stock (or our Vegetable Stock, previous recipe)
- 1 tablespoon Crushed Red Pepper Flakes
- 1 1/2 tablespoon Pure Honey

Salt & Fresh Cracked Black Pepper T.T.

Directions:

1. **Heat medium cast iron pan**, and add in 1 tablespoon of your grapeseed oil. Once your oil is hot add in your uncut tomatoes and uncut garlic cloves. Season with salt and roast all sides of the tomatoes and garlic evenly. This step is crucial to the "roasted garlic flavor".
2. **To a medium sauce pot**, add in your roasted tomatoes, roasted garlic, remaining 3 tablespoons of grapeseed oil, dried basil, dried oregano, kale stock, red pepper flakes and honey and simmer together on medium low heat.
3. **Next,** you'll either need to blend everything in a stand blender or you can leave it in the sauce pot and use an emulsifying hand blender.
4. **Add** salt and fresh cracked black pepper to taste.
5. **Serve with** garlic bread or make homemade pizzas or flatbreads using this sauce or store in an air tight container in the fridge or freezer. Reheat this sauce in a sauce pan on low heat until aromatic and saucy.

How To Infuse: Either add in cannabis infused tincture or sub the grapeseed oil for cannabis infused grapeseed oil being sure to watch the overall dosage of the sauce.
Variation: If you're not a fan of honey, switch it out for pure agave or pure maple syrup which you can also use to infuse with.

Presto Pesto Sauce

You do not have to have pecans or Parmesan cheese to make this amazing pesto sauce. The roasted pecans are left in there because traditionally it's made with pine nuts, but we like the crunch factor and the nuttiness that pecans provide to the pesto.

Prep Time: 30 Minutes
Oven Time: 10 Minutes

Infusion Options:
Cannabis Tincture, Cooking Oil
Decarboxylated Flower/Kief

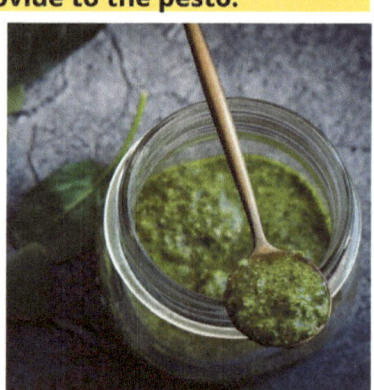

When it comes to the Parmesan cheese, you can make this recipe vegan by using alternative cheeses from brands like Follow Your Heart or Miyoko's or just anything that fits your taste buds. Have it your way!

Ingredients:

- 1 cup Kale, Washed
- 2 each Garlic Cloves
- 1/2 each Lemon Juice
- 1/4 cup Fresh Cilantro & Fresh Scallion
- 1/4 cup Roasted Pecans (optional)
- 1 cup Garlic Oil (or olive oil)
- 1/2 cup Parmesan Cheese (optional)
- Salt & Fresh Cracked Black Pepper T.T.

Directions:

1. **First, put your pecans** in the oven at 350° they should take about 10 minutes or until you start to smell that it's roasted
2. **Next, you're going to wash** your kale, half will be cooked and the other you're going to keep raw
3. **Once the Kale is cooked** and the other is washed, dry your kale before you add into the blender with two cloves of garlic, half squeeze a lemon, and a fourth a cup of cilantro and scallions
4. **Add a fourth a cup of garlic oil** and turn the blender on and from here on out you're going to gradually add in the rest of your oil. You want to make sure your pesto consistency is a bit loose when done.
5. **Once you like the consistency** of your pesto pour into another container and add in your Parmesan cheese.
6. **Presto We Have Pesto!** Serve with fresh vegetable tray, chicken wings or use in your favorite pasta or steak recipe.

How To Infuse: Add your favorite dose of tincture, infused cooking oil or activated ground flower/kief for your own portion or enough to serve the group. Our recommended single dose is any where between 10mg to 25mg per person.

Oven Roasted Tomato Sauce

Homemade fire oven roasted tomatoes from on the vine is really and truly something special, especially if you own a gas oven or an awesome brick/wooden/electric fire pit/oven. If you don't, follow step one from making our Garlic Roasted Pizza Sauce recipe.

Prep Time: 10 Minutes
Cook Time: 2 Hours
Yield: Appx. 2 Cups

Infusion Options:
Cannabis Tincture or Cannabis Oil

Ingredients:

- 8 each Tomatoes On The Vine, Uncut
- 3 each Fresh Garlic Cloves, Diced
- 1 each Medium White Onion, Diced
- 1 sprig Fresh Tarragon
- 1 sprig Fresh Rosemary
- 1 sprig Fresh Oregano
- 4 sprigs Fresh Thyme
- 5 each Fresh Basil Leaves
- 1 tablespoon Grapeseed Oil
- 1/2 cup Vegetable Stock (see page 27)
- 1 teaspoon Whole Cloves
- 1 each Star Anise
- 1/2 tablespoon Crushed Red Pepper Flakes

Salt & Fresh Cracked Black Pepper T.T.

Directions:

1. **First, put your tomatoes** drizzles with a little grapeseed oil and salt in the oven at 400°. They should take about 10 minutes caramelize or until you start to smell that it's roasted.
2. **To a medium sauce pot,** add in the diced garlic, diced onion and caramelize with a tablespoon of grapeseed oil until translucent. this
3. **Once caramelized,** and in the roasted tomatoes, tarragon, rosemary, oregano, thyme, basil, red pepper flakes, whole cloves, star anise and vegetable stock and simmer together on medium low heat.
4. **Next,** you'll either need to blend everything in a stand blender or you can leave it in the sauce pot and use an emulsifying hand blender.
5. **Add** salt and fresh cracked black pepper to taste.
6. **Serve** with garlic bread or make spagetti using this sauce or store in an air tight container in the fridge or freezer. Reheat this sauce in a sauce pan on low heat until aromatic and saucy.

How To Infuse: Add in cannabis infused tincture or cannabis oil being sure to watch the overall dosage of the sauce.

Soup & Salads

59	Broccoli, Cauliflower & Cheddar Soup
60	Hot Kale Salad
61	Vegan Caesar Salad
62	White Chicken Chili Soup

The beauty in soup is you can enjoy it more often than just from a cold or as an appetizer. You can easily pair soup with your choice of bread or even side by side with a salad.

As far a salad goes, it is enjoyable throughout the day. Make it a heartier salad by adding any meat protein or vegan protein of your choice to bulk it up.

Broccoli, Cauliflower & Cheddar Soup

This soup reminds me of home and comfort but it is more than that because it's also versatile. Have you ever had broccoli and cheddar dip? Well the those two recipes are basically the same. Our version of the classic recipe also contains cauliflower which is equally as much important to us as broccoli.

Prep Time: 30 Minutes
Cook Time: 1 Hour
Yield: 4 to 6 Servings

Infusion Options:
Cannabis Tincture or Cannabis Butter or Cannabis Oil

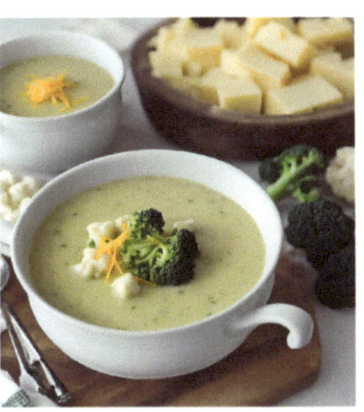

Ingredients:

- 1/2 stick Unsalted Butter, Room Temperature
- 1 medium White Onion, Diced
- 3 each Fresh Garlic Cloves, Diced
- 4 tablespoons Unbleached All-Purpose Flour
- 2 1/2 cups Vegetable Stock (see page 24)
- 1 Broccoli Head Chopped Into Florets
- 1 Cauliflower Head Chopped Into Florets
- 1 medium Carrot, Diced or Shredded
- 16 ounces Heavy Cream or Full-Fat Coconut Cream
- 8 ounces Cheddar Cheese
- 4 tablespoons Nutritional Yeast
- 1 tablespoon Smoked Paprika
- 1 tablespoon Crushed Red Pepper Flakes, Optional
- 4 sprigs Fresh Thyme

Salt & Fresh Cracked Black Pepper T.T.

To make this recipe vegan:
sub vegan butter, sub vegan cheddar cheese & use full-fat coconut cream
Pro Tip: Remember to save your scraps..

Directions:

1. **In a large dutch oven or stock pot,** melt the butter on medium to high heat.
2. **Add the diced onions** and cook 3-4 minutes or until its a golden caramel color and the smell is very aromatic. Then add in your diced garlic and sauté for another minute.
3. **Next, add in the flour** and whisk for 1-2 minutes or until the flour begins to turn golden in color. This is called your rue. Pour in the vegetable stock, broccoli florets, cauliflower florets, carrots, and seasoning.
4. **Bring to a boil,** add in the fresh thyme, reduce heat to medium-low and simmer for 15 minutes or until the broccoli and carrots are cooked through.
5. **Stir in heavy cream or coconut cream** and cheddar cheese and simmer for another few minutes. Taste and adjust seasoning if needed.
6. **Serve with** toasted crusty bread or in a bread bowl if desired.

How To Infuse: Add in cannabis infused tincture, cannabis oil or cannabis butter being sure to watch the overall dosage of the soup.

Hot Kale Salad

This salad is great for a quick and hot meal. There simply is not another salad like this one. Experience kale in a new way with our quick and easy salad that is both great for everyday healthly meals and on-the-go lunches.

Prep Time: 15 Minutes
Cook Time: 15 Minutes
Yield: 1 to 2 Servings

Infusion Options:
Cannabis Tincture or Cannabis Oil

Ingredients:

- 2 tablespoons Grapeseed Oil or Butter
- 1/2 small Sweet Red Onion, Sliced
- 1 each Fresh Garlic Clove, Diced
- 1/2 can Chick Peas, Drained
- 1/4 cup Gourmet Mushroom Blend, Sliced
- 1 bunch Chopped Kale
- 1 bunch Baby Spinach, Optional
- 1 teaspoon Smoked Paprika
- 1/2 teaspoon Crushed Red Pepper Flakes, Optional

For Topping:
- Toasted Almonds
- Dried Cranberries

Balsamic Glaze, To Drizzle
Salt & Fresh Cracked Black Pepper T.T.

There's so many ways you can mix this recipe up. You can add chicken, tofu or shrimp. But trust you'll want to keep that balance of balsamic, cranberries & almonds. It is truly harmonious!

Directions:

1. **Heat a medium sauté pan ,** with grapeseed oil on medium heat.
2. **Add the diced onions** and cook 3-4 minutes or until its a golden caramel color and the smell is very aromatic. Then add in your diced garlic and sauté for another minute.
3. **Next, add in the chick peas,** mushrooms and add in all of your seasonings. You want the chick peas to be lightly toasted and evenly coated in the pan.
4. **Now add in your greens,** this part is really quick so make sure to keep your pan moving while stirring the ingredients in the pan with a rubber spatula. As soon as your green start to wilt, turn off the heat.
5. Drizzle on as much balsamic glaze as you like and add in your almonds and cranberries. Toss this togetherin the pan once more without heat.
6. **Serve immediately or pack it to go.**

How To Infuse: Cook this quick salad with cannabis oil or top with cannabis tincture once your salad is ready.

Vegan Caesar Salad

This caesar salad is so special and so dear to us because the recipe is adapted from our Aunt Karen. This recipe is vegan but of course add chicken if you want!

Prep Time: 20 Minutes
Cook Time: 45 Minutes
Yield: 6 to 8 Servings

**Infusion Options:
Cannabis Tincture or Cannabis Oil**

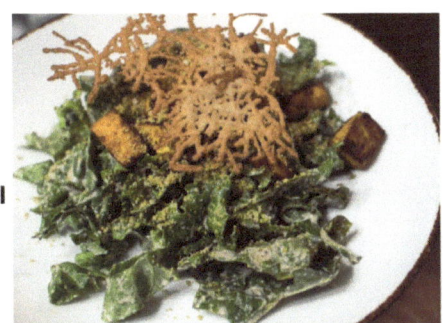

Ingredients:

For The Tofu:
- 1 pressed Extra Firm Tofu Block, Cut Into Cubes
- 1 tablespoon Light Brown Sugar
- 1 teaspoon Ground Smoked Paprika
- 1/2 teaspoon Ground Ginger
- 1/2 teaspoon Ground Turmeric
- 1/2 teaspoon Coriander Seeds
- 1 teaspoon Crushed Red Chili Flakes
- 2 tablespoons Cornstarch

For The Topping:
- 4 ounces Unsalted Cashews
- 1 teaspoon Garlic Powder
- 2 tablespoons Nutritional Yeast
- 3 tablespoons Hemp Seeds
- 2 each Garlic Cloves

For The Caesar Dressing:
- 16 ounces Unsalted Cashews, Soaked
- Extra Virgin Olive Oil
- Lemon Juice & Zest
- 1 tablespoon Dijon Mustard
- 1/2 each Cucumber, Chopped
- 2 teaspoons Garlic Powder
- 1 tablespoon Liquid Smoke
- 1 tablespoon Capers
- 1 teaspoon Dried or Fresh Oregano

For The Salad:
- Romaine Lettuce

Top with Vegan Parmesan Cheese
Salt & Fresh Cracked Black Pepper T.T.

Directions:

1. **For the tofu,** season with brown sugar, smoked paprika, ginger, turmeric, coriander, crushed red chili flakes, cornstarch and let marinate. While that's marinating get your sautee pan or cast iron skillet nice and hot.
2. **When your pan is hot,** add in a little oil to coat the pan. Next, sear the tofu on all sides until evenly golden brown. Top with fresh salt and pepper.
3. **For the topping,** blend the cashews, garlic cloves, garlic powder, nutritional yeast and hemp seed with salt and pepper to taste until you have a fine crumbly texture.
4. **For the caesar dressing,** once your cashews are soaked, blend them along with olive oil, lemon juice, lemon zest, dijon mustard, garlic powder, liquid smoke, capers, oregano along with fresh salt and pepper to taste until creamy and smooth.
5. **Wash your romaine lettuce** and chop to your desired size. Toss the lettuce in the dressing and finish it with the topping, tofu and parmesan cheese.
6. **Enjoy**!

How To Infuse: Add in cannabis infused tincture or cannabis oil to the dressing recipe being sure to watch the overall dosage for each portion. Side Note: If you're not vegan, just sub for real cheese and a meat protein.

White Chicken Chili Soup

This recipe is home as it takes quite a bit of time to make but so worth it in the end. Pair this recipe with one of our bread recipes & you're set!

Prep Time: 45 Minutes
Cook Time: 1 Hour
Yield: 6 to 8 Servings

Infusion Options:
Cannabis Tincture or Cannabis Butter or Cannabis Oil

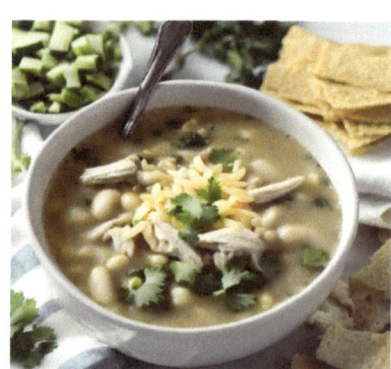

Ingredients:

- 2-16 ounce cans White Northern Beans
- 1 medium White Onion, Sliced
- 1 stick Unsalted Butter, Made To Browned Butter)
- 4 tablespoons Unbleached All-Purpose Flour
- 6 ounces Chicken Broth
- 16 ounces Half & Half
- 1 tablespoon Tabasco Hot Sauce
- 1 1/2 teaspoons Ground Chili Powder
- 1 teaspoon Ground Cumin
- 4 ounces Diced Jalapeños with Juice
- 2 to 4 Boneless Organic Chicken Breast
- Monterey Jack Cheese
- Sour Cream
- 4 sprigs Fresh Thyme

Salt & Fresh Cracked Black Pepper T.T.

Directions:

1. **Heat a large skillet** over moderately high heat and put in some butter and oil.
2. **Meanwhile,** coat the chicken with some salt, pepper and chili powder. Throw them in the skillet - Leave them for 5 minutes or until nicely brown, then flip them. Leave it there until browned and then flip them every few minutes until they are done. I usually cook them 80%- they'll finish in the stew.
3. **When the chicken is cool enough to handle,** shred it with your fingers and set aside. While waiting for the chicken to cool, cook the chopped onion in the same pan with 2 Tbs. of butter until softened.
4. **In a heavy soup pot,** large enough to hold all the ingredients melt the remaining 6 Tbs. of butter over moderately low heat and whisk in flour. Cook the roux, whisking constantly for 3 minutes. Stir in the onion and gradually add the broth and the half and half, whisking the whole time.
5. **Bring the mixture to a boil and simmer,** stirring occasionally, 5 minutes, or until thickened. Stir in Tabasco, chili powder, cumin, salt and pepper. Add beans with the liquid, chilies with the liquid, chicken and cheese, and cook over moderately low heat, stirring occasionally for 20 minutes. Stir in sour cream.
6. **May be served immediately** – though like all chilies this tastes awesome the next day! • Serve with the usual chili garnishes – cilantro, cheese, chopped jalapeños, tomatoes, corn bread, etc.

How To Infuse: Add in cannabis infused tincture, cannabis oil or cannabis butter being sure to watch the overall dosage for each portion.

Appetizers

64	Cauliflower Bites
65	Fancy Avocado Toast
66	Game Day Chicken Wings
67	Quick Flatbread Pizza
68	Truffle Honey Potato Fries

Appetizers are truly underrated. These are basically bite size entrees doing the most. The beauty of them, is that appetizers have the ability to be versatile. They can serve as a passed hors d'oeuvres or as a tapa.

This is your favorite munchie section. No party is a party without any of our infused appetizer bites.

Cauliflower Bites

This recipe is perfectly roasted and deliciously seasoned, these bite-sized delights offer a tasty and healthier snack alternative that you won't be able to resist.

Prep Time: 15 Minutes
Bake Time: 25 Minutes
Yield: 4 Servings

Infusion Option:
Cannabis Tincture, Cannabis Oil

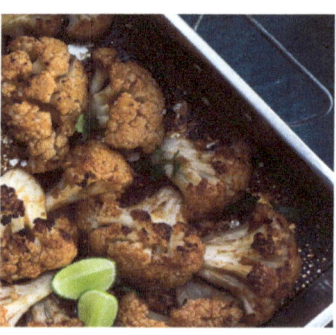

Ingredients:

- 1 large Cauliflower Head
- 1 cup All-Purpose Flour (or gluten-free flour for a gluten-free option)
- 1 teaspoon Garlic Powder
- 1 teaspoon Paprika
- 1 cup Milk (or non-dairy milk for a vegan option)
- 1 cup Breadcrumbs (or gluten-free breadcrumbs for a gluten-free option)

Salt & Fresh Cracked Black Pepper T.T.

Directions:

1. **Preheat the oven.** Preheat your oven to 425°F (220°C). Line a baking sheet with parchment paper or lightly grease it with cooking spray or oil.
2. **Prepare the cauliflower.** Cut the cauliflower into bite-sized florets, discarding the tough stem. Wash and thoroughly dry the florets.
3. **Prepare the breading station.** In three separate bowls, set up a breading station. In the first bowl, combine the flour, garlic powder, paprika, salt, and black pepper. In the second bowl, pour the milk. In the third bowl, place the breadcrumbs.
4. **Bread the cauliflower.** Take a cauliflower floret and dip it into the flour mixture, making sure it's evenly coated. Shake off any excess flour. Then, dip the floret into the milk, allowing any excess to drip off. Finally, roll the floret in the breadcrumbs, pressing gently to adhere the breadcrumbs. Place the coated floret on the prepared baking sheet. Repeat the process for the remaining florets.
5. **Bake the cauliflower bites.** Once all the florets are coated and on the baking sheet, lightly spray or drizzle them with cooking spray or oil to help them crisp up. Bake in the preheated oven for about 20-25 minutes, or until the cauliflower is tender and the coating is golden brown and crispy.
6. **Serve and enjoy.** Serve the cauliflower bites as a tasty appetizer or snack. They can be enjoyed on their own or with your favorite dipping sauce like buffalo or sweet chili.

Fancy Avocado Toast

Absolutely anyone can make this recipe. It's perfect for on-the-go mornings, brunch or late lunches. But this recipe is fancy enough to pass for an amazing light pizza for dinner.

Prep Time: 20+ Minutes
Yield: 2 to 4 Servings

Infusion Option:
Cannabis Tincture or Cannabis Oil or Cannabis Butter

Ingredients:

- 4 slices Bread of Choice
- 2 each Ripe Avocado, Lightly Smashed or Sliced

Topping Options:
- Sun-Dried Tomatoes
- Cherry Tomatoes
- Crispy Applewood Smoked Bacon
- Sauteed Mushrooms
- Sliced Jalapeños
- Drizzled Honey
- Drizzled Balsamic Glaze
- Fried Sunny Side Up Eggs
- Smoked Salmon, Thinly Sliced
- Capers
- Truffle Butter
- Grilled Shredded Chicken
- Dried Fruit
- Figs, Sliced
- Nuts and/or Seeds

Smoked Paprika, Salt & Fresh Cracked Black Pepper T.T.

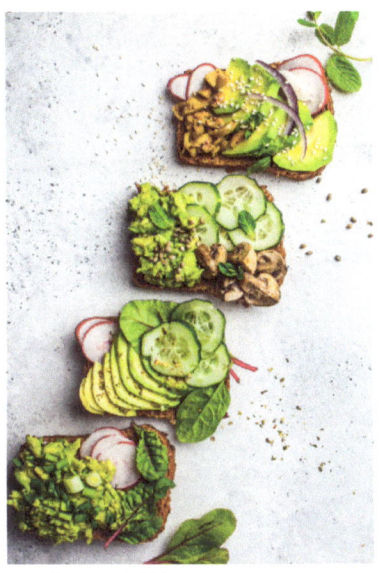

- Chopped Chives
- Chopped Basil
- Chopped Cilantro
- Pickled Onions
- Garlic Powder
- Kalamata Olives
- Microgreens
- Roasted Chick Peas or Beans
- Radishes, Thinly Sliced

Directions:

1. **First,** by no mean necessary do you have to use every single topping listed above. Have fun with it or use what you already have at home. If there's an ingredient you don't see listed above that you'd like to add, go ahead and get fancy.
2. **Begin by toasting** your choice of bread first. Then add avocado and all of your toppings.
3. **For pizza variation,** either buy premade flat bread or pizza dough. If using flat bread, toast it first just like the sliced bread. If using pizza dough, roll out and bake until toasted golden.
4. **Enjoy this however you like!**

How To Infuse: Add in cannabis infused tincture, cannabis oil or cannabis butter being sure to watch the overall dosage for each portion.

Game Day Chicken Wings

Not just for game day but still perfect for when the day comes! This recipe is quick and easy to make and a definite crowd pleaser!

Prep Time: 30 Minutes
Bake Time: 25 Minutes
Yield: 6 Servings

Infusion Option:
Cannabis Honey, Cannabis Oil

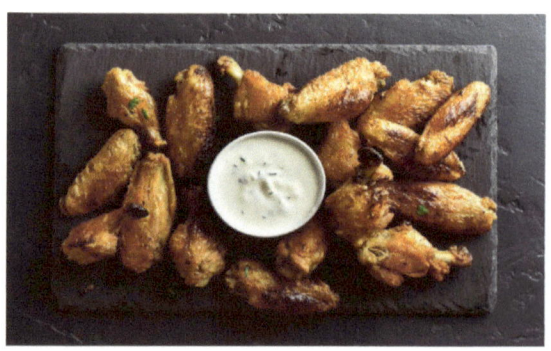

Ingredients:

- 2 pounds Chicken Wings
- ¼ cup Honey
- 3 tablespoons Soy Sauce
- 3 tablespoons Hot Sauce (adjust according to your spice preference)
- 3 cloves Garlic, minced
- 1 teaspoon Ginger, grated
- 1 tablespoon Olive Oil
- Chopped Green Onions and Sesame Seeds for garnish (optional)

Salt & Fresh Cracked Black Pepper T.T.

Directions:

1. Preheat the oven to 425°F (220°C) and line a baking sheet with parchment paper.
2. In a bowl, combine honey, soy sauce, hot sauce, minced garlic, grated ginger, olive oil, salt, and pepper. Mix well to create the sauce.
3. Place the chicken wings in a large bowl and pour half of the sauce over them. Toss the wings until they are evenly coated.
4. Arrange the wings in a single layer on the prepared baking sheet. Reserve the remaining sauce for later.
5. Bake the chicken wings in the preheated oven for 40-45 minutes, flipping them halfway through, until they are golden brown and crispy.
6. While the wings are baking, heat the reserved sauce in a small saucepan over medium heat. Simmer for a few minutes until it thickens slightly.
7. Once the wings are cooked, remove them from the oven and brush them with the heated sauce.
8. Return the wings to the oven for an additional 5 minutes to allow the sauce to caramelize.
9. Remove the wings from the oven and let them cool slightly.
10. **Garnish** with chopped green onions and sesame seeds, if desired.

Quick Flatbread Pizza

It's really easy to have fun with recipe and make it your own. Like our recipe for the vegetable stock or avocado toast, you can use whatever ingredients you're in the mood for or have stocked in your kitchen.

Prep Time: 20 Minutes
Yield: 2 to 4 Servings

Infusion Option:
Cannabis Tincture or Cannabis Oil or Cannabis Butter

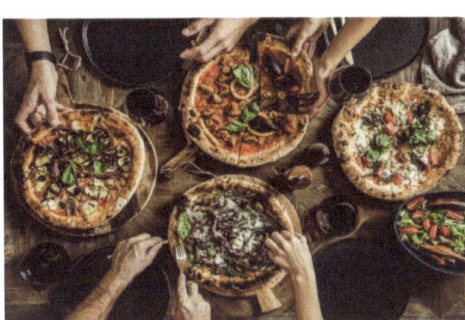

Ingredients:

Choose your flatbread:
- Naan Bread

OR Pita Bread
OR our pizza dough recipe (rolled thinner for flatbread variation)

Choose your sauce:
- Brown Butter Alfredo Sauce, for a white sauce flatbread

OR Garlic Roasted Pizza Sauce, for traditional flatbread
OR Pesto Sauce, for less traditional

Choose your toppings:
- Veggies of your choice
- Meat of your choice, if vegan, use plant-based options
- Cheeses of your choice, yes use at least two!

But don't go without these finishers:
- 1 Extra Virgin Olive Oil, for garnish to drizzle

Salt & Fresh Cracked Black Pepper T.T.

Directions:

1. **Preheat your oven to 350 degrees Fahrenheit.**
2. **Toast** your choice of flatbread first. If using pizza dough, roll out thin and bake until toasted golden.
3. **Add** your sauce of choice.
4. **Layer on toppings.** Then add cheese and all of your toppings.
5. **Bake.** Pop it all back in the oven for about 10 to 15 minutes or until it's baked the way you like it.
6. **Remove from oven.** Garnish finished flatbread with extra virgin olive oil, salt and fresh cracked black pepper.

Truffle Honey Potato Fries

Delight in our Truffle Honey Potato Fries, where every bite offers a sweet crunch. Perfect as an appetizer or a quick snack, these indulgent treats will have you hooked from the first taste!

Prep Time: 20 Minutes
Cook Time: 30 Minutes
Yield: 2 to 4 Servings

Infusion Option:
Cannabis Honey or Cannabis Oil

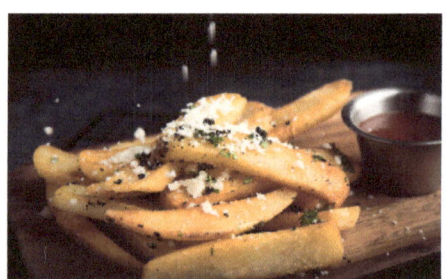

Ingredients:

- 1 pound Russet Potatoes
- 2 tablespoons Olive Oil
- 2 tablespoons Truffle Oil (good quality, not essence or artificially flavored)
- 2 tablespoons Honey
- Fresh Parsley, chopped (for garnish, optional)

Salt & Fresh Cracked Black Pepper T.T.

Directions:

1. **Preheat the oven.** Preheat your oven to 425°F (220°C). Line a baking sheet with parchment paper or lightly grease it with cooking spray.
2. **Prepare the potatoes.** Wash the potatoes and pat them dry. Leave the skins on for added texture and flavor. Cut the potatoes into fry shaped pieces, ensuring they are relatively uniform in size for even cooking.
3. **Toss with olive oil and seasonings.** In a large bowl, toss the potato pieces with olive oil until they are well coated. Season with salt and pepper to taste. Mix well to ensure the seasoning is evenly distributed.
4. **Roast the potatoes.** Spread the seasoned potato pieces in a single layer on the prepared baking sheet. Roast in the preheated oven for about 25-30 minutes or until the potatoes are golden brown and crispy, flipping them halfway through the cooking time for even browning.
5. **Prepare the truffle honey glaze.** In a small bowl, whisk together the truffle oil and honey until well combined.
6. **Toss the potatoes in the glaze.** Once the potatoes are cooked, transfer them to a large mixing bowl. Drizzle the truffle honey glaze over the hot potatoes and toss gently to coat them evenly.
7. **Garnish and serve.** Sprinkle the truffle honey potato bites with fresh chopped parsley, if desired, for added freshness and presentation. Serve them immediately as an appetizer or a flavorful side dish.

Side Dishes

70   Candied Sweet Potato Mash
71   Garlic & Herb Baked Potatoes
72   Maple Bacon Brussel Sprouts
73   Truffle Mac & Cheese

Side dishes make perfect appetizers as well. And also, carbs are great. Don't let anyone tell you otherwise. We live for carbs in this house. That's it, that's all!

Candied Sweet Potato Mash

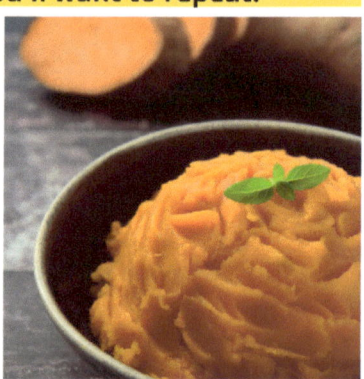

Add a dash of festive flavor to your holiday spread with our Candied Sweet Potato Mash. Its sweet, caramelized goodness pairs perfectly with your celebratory feasts, making it a tradition you'll want to repeat.

Prep Time: 15 Minutes
Cook Time: 45+ Minutes
Yield: 4 Servings

Infusion Option:
Cannabis Maple Syrup or Cannabis Butter

Ingredients:

- 3 large Sweet Potatoes
- 1/4 cup Unsalted Butter, melted
- 1/4 cup Brown Sugar
- 1/4 cup Maple Syrup
- 1/4 cup Heavy Cream (or substitute for non-dairy alternative like coconut cream)
- 1/2 teaspoon Ground Cinnamon
- 1/4 teaspoon Ground Nutmeg
- Fresh Parsley, chopped (for garnish, optional)

Salt & Fresh Cracked Black Pepper T.T.

Directions:

1. **Preheat the oven.** Preheat your oven to 375°F (190°C).
2. **Prepare the sweet potatoes.** Wash the sweet potatoes and pat them dry. Pierce each sweet potato several times with a fork to allow steam to escape during baking. Place the sweet potatoes on a baking sheet lined with foil or parchment paper.
3. **Bake the sweet potatoes.** Place the baking sheet with the sweet potatoes in the preheated oven and bake for about 45-60 minutes, or until the sweet potatoes are tender when pierced with a fork. The baking time may vary depending on the size of the sweet potatoes. Remove them from the oven and let them cool for a few minutes.
4. **Prepare the candied mixture.** Peel the baked sweet potatoes and place the flesh in a large mixing bowl. Mash the sweet potatoes with a potato masher or fork until smooth. Add melted butter, brown sugar, maple syrup, heavy cream, cinnamon, nutmeg, and salt to the mashed sweet potatoes. Mix well until all the ingredients are fully combined.
5. **Transfer to a baking dish.** Grease a baking dish with butter. Transfer the sweet potato mixture to the prepared baking dish, spreading it evenly.
6. **Serve and enjoy.** Remove the candied sweet potato mash from the oven. Allow it to cool for a few minutes before serving.

Garlic & Herb Baked Potatoes

These twice baked garlic and herb stuffed potatoes with cheese offer a flavorful twist on traditional mashed potatoes, with the added goodness of crispy potato skins.

Prep Time: 20 Minutes
Bake Time: 15 Minutes
Yield: 4 Servings

Infusion Option:
Cannabis Maple Syrup or Cannabis Butter

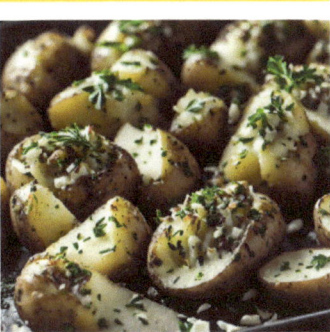

Ingredients:

- 4 large Russet Potatoes
- 4 cloves Garlic, Minced
- 1/2 cup Unsalted Butter, Melted
- 1/2 cup Milk (or more as needed for desired consistency)
- 1 cup Shredded Cheddar Cheese (or your preferred cheese)
- 2 tablespoons Fresh Herbs (such as parsley, chives, or thyme), finely chopped

Salt & Fresh Cracked Black Pepper T.T.

Directions:

1. **Preheat the oven.** Preheat your oven to 400°F (200°C).
2. **Prepare the potatoes.** Scrub the potatoes thoroughly to remove any dirt. Leave the skin on for added texture and flavor. Pat the potatoes dry.
3. **Pierce the potatoes.** Use a fork to poke several holes in each potato to allow steam to escape while baking.
4. **Bake the potatoes.** Place the potatoes directly on the oven rack or on a baking sheet. Bake for about 50-60 minutes, or until the potatoes are tender when pierced with a fork.
5. **Prepare the filling.** While the potatoes are baking, in a small bowl, mix together the minced garlic, melted butter, shredded cheese, fresh herbs, salt, and pepper. Set the mixture aside.
6. **Slice and scoop.** Once the potatoes are baked and slightly cooled, slice them in half lengthwise. Using a spoon, scoop out the potato flesh into a large mixing bowl, leaving a thin layer of potato attached to the skin for stability.
7. **Mash and mix.** Mash the potato flesh with a fork or potato masher until desired consistency. Add the prepared garlic and herb filling mixture to the mashed potatoes and stir to combine. Gradually pour in the milk while stirring until the desired creamy consistency is reached. Adjust the seasoning with salt and pepper to taste.
8. **Fill the potato skins.** Spoon the mashed potato mixture back into the potato skins, dividing it evenly among them.
9. **Bake and broil.** Place the filled potato skins on a baking sheet and return them to the oven. Bake for about 10-15 minutes, or until the tops are golden brown. For an extra crispy top, turn on the broiler for the last few minutes, keeping a close eye to prevent burning. Serve when ready.

Maple Bacon Brussel Sprouts

==The combination of the sweet maple syrup, tangy balsamic vinegar, smoky bacon, and caramelized Brussels sprouts creates a flavorful and satisfying dish.==

Prep Time: 20 Minutes
Cook Time: 25 Minutes
Yield: 4 Servings

Infusion Option:
Cannabis Maple Syrup or Cannabis Oil

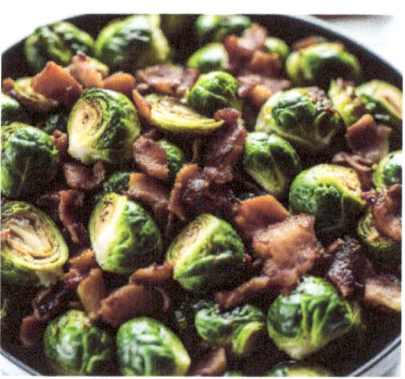

Ingredients:

- 1/2 pound Brussels Sprouts, Trimmed and Halved
- 6 slices Bacon, Sliced to Pieces
- 2 tablespoons Maple Syrup
- 2 tablespoons Balsamic Vinegar
- 2 tablespoons Olive Oil
- 1/2 teaspoon Garlic Powder
- 1/2 teaspoon Smoked Paprika

Salt & Fresh Cracked Black Pepper T.T.

Directions:

1. **Preheat the oven.** Preheat your oven to 425°F (220°C).
2. **Prepare the Brussels sprouts.** Trim the ends of the Brussel sprouts and cut them in half lengthwise. Remove any loose outer leaves.
3. **Cook the bacon.** In a skillet over medium heat, cook the bacon until crispy. Once cooked, remove the bacon from the skillet and let it cool. Crumble the bacon into small pieces.
4. **Make the glaze.** In a small bowl, whisk together the maple syrup, balsamic vinegar, olive oil, garlic powder, smoked paprika, salt, and pepper until well combined.
5. **Toss the Brussels sprouts.** Place the halved Brussels sprouts in a large mixing bowl. Pour the glaze over the Brussels sprouts and toss to coat them evenly.
6. **Roast the Brussels sprouts**. Spread the coated Brussels sprouts in a single layer on a baking sheet lined with parchment paper. Place the baking sheet in the preheated oven and roast for about 20-25 minutes, or until the Brussels sprouts are tender and caramelized, stirring halfway through the cooking time for even browning.
7. **Add the bacon.** Remove the Brussels sprouts from the oven and sprinkle the crumbled bacon over the top.
8. **Serve and enjoy!**

Truffle Mac & Cheese

This truffle mac and cheese recipe combines the richness of smoked gouda, manchego, and cheddar cheese with the earthy flavor of truffle oil, resulting in a decadent and flavorful dish.

Prep Time: 20 Minutes
Cook Time: 40 Minutes
Yield: 4 Servings

Infusion Option:
Cannabis Maple Butter, Cannabis Oil

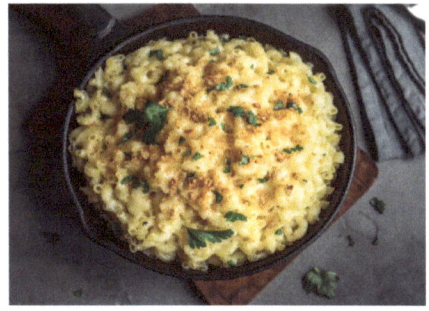

Ingredients:

- 12 ounces Pipe Rigate Pasta Noodles
- 4 tablespoons Unsalted Butter
- 1/4 cup All-Purpose Flour
- 2 cups Whole Milk
- 1 cup Heavy Cream
- 8 ounces Smoked Gouda Cheese, gGated
- 4 ounces Manchego Cheese, Grated
- 4 ounces Sharp Cheddar Cheese, Grated
- 1 tablespoon Truffle Oil (again, authentic)
- 1/2 teaspoon Garlic Powder
- 1/2 teaspoon Onion Powder
- 1/2 teaspoon Smoked Paprika
- 1/2 teaspoon Dried Oregano
- Chopped Fresh Parsley for garnish (optional)
- Salt & Fresh Cracked Black Pepper T.T.

Directions:

1. **Cook the pasta.** Cook the pipe rigate pasta according to the package instructions until al dente. Drain and set aside.
2. **Preheat the oven.** Preheat your oven to 375°F (190°C).
3. **Prepare the cheese sauce.** In a large saucepan, melt the butter over medium heat. Add the flour and whisk constantly for about 1-2 minutes until a roux forms. Gradually pour in the milk and heavy cream, whisking continuously to prevent lumps. Cook the mixture for about 5 minutes, or until it thickens.
4. **Add the cheeses.** Reduce the heat to low and gradually add the grated smoked gouda, manchego, and cheddar cheese to the sauce, stirring until melted and smooth. Reserve a small portion of each cheese for topping and layering. Stir in the truffle oil, garlic powder, onion powder, smoked paprika, dried oregano, salt, and pepper to taste. Continue to heat the sauce until all the cheeses are fully melted and the flavors are well combined.
5. **Combine the pasta and cheese sauce.** Add the cooked pipe rigate pasta to the cheese sauce, tossing gently until the pasta is fully coated.
6. **Transfer to a baking dish.** Pour the mac and cheese mixture into a greased baking dish making sure to layer additional cheese halfway through. Then sprinkle a little more grated cheeses on top for an extra cheesy crust.
7. **Bake the mac and cheese.** Place the baking dish in the preheated oven and bake for 20-25 minutes, or until the top is golden and bubbly.
8. **Garnish and serve.** Remove the truffle mac and cheese from the oven and let it cool slightly. Garnish with chopped fresh parsley, if desired, for a pop of color and freshness. Serve hot and enjoy!

Main Dish

75	Brown Butter Alfredo Pasta
76	Creamy Spinach Rotini
77	Pan Seared Caulifower
78	Portobello Mushroom Burger
79	Truffle Honey Mushroom Pasta

Main dishes are the main event, especially if you're looking empress your family and friends with an infused meal! As with the rest of the book, have fun with this chapter. Make substitutions, swap out proteins, get creative. The possibilities are endless!

Now that you've made it to this chapter, you're well on your way to understandin how to infuse different types of food using different mediums.

Brown Butter Alfredo Pasta

> As we've stated before, this recipe is home for us. Pair our Brown Butter Alfredo Sauce to easily make this recipe. The sauce itself can be stored in a container and refrigerated for up to 1 week. Serve with a cooked vegetable or protein of your choice. We like cavatappi pasta paired with pan seared chicken breast finished with parmesan crisps.

Prep Time: 5 Minutes
Cook Time: 15 Minutes
Yield: 4 Servings

Infusion Options:
Cannabis Butter or Cannabis Tincture or Cannabis Oil

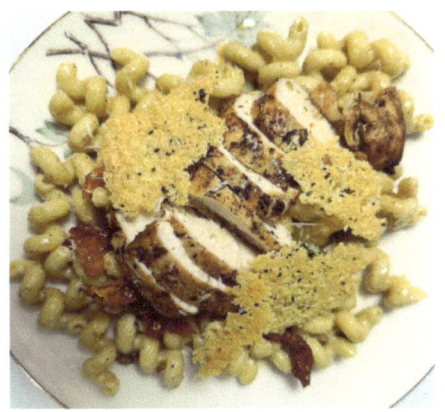

Ingredients:

- Brown Butter Alfredo Sauce
- 8 ounces Pasta (of your choice)
- 2 tablespoons Unsalted Butter

Garnish with Sun Dried Tomatoes (Optional)
Salt & Fresh Cracked Black Pepper T.T.

Directions:

1. **Start** by heating a medium saute pan on medium to high heat. While that is heating, add water to a stock pot with kosher salt for the pasta.
2. **Once your sauté pan is hot,** add in your already made Alfredo sauce to heat it up. Use as much or as little as you like depending on how saucy you would like the outcome of the dish to be. Reduce to low heat.
3. **In the meantime,** boil the pasta until it is al dente which means just barely undercooked. This is a chefs tip as to not end up with mushy pasta in the end.
4. **With your now ready pasta,** coat in butter and season with fresh black pepper.
5. **On low heat,** mix in your pasta until it is fully coated in the brown butter Alfredo sauce. If you would like to thin out the sauce, add in a bit of pasta water.
6. **Serve right away** finished with fresh cracked black pepper and top with additional parmesan cheese.

> **How To Infuse:** Add in cannabis infused tincture, cannabis oil or cannabis butter being sure to watch the overall dosage for each portion.

Creamy Spinach Rotini

For the record, this recipe would also make for a fantastic ravioli if you're up for all of the prep that goes along with making that version of this recipe. We encourage you to get creative and have fun!

Prep Time: 5 Minutes
Cook Time: 15 Minutes
Yield: 4 Servings

Infusion Options:
Cannabis Butter or Cannabis Tincture or Cannabis Oil

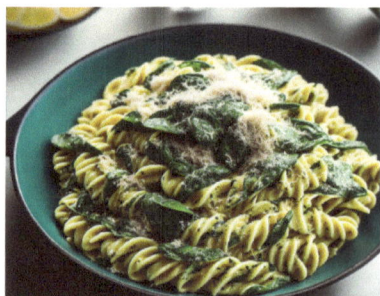

Ingredients:

- Brown Butter Alfredo Sauce, previous recipe
- 8 ounces Rotini Pasta
- 2 tablespoons Unsalted Butter
- 8 ounces Vegan Miyoko's Savory Scallion Cream Cheese
- 2 cups Spinach
- 1 each Yellow Bell Pepper
- 2 cloves Fresh Garlic, Minced
- 1 teaspoon Italian Seasoning
- 1/2 teaspoon Garlic Powder
- 1/2 teaspoon Onion Powder
- Salt & Fresh Cracked Black Pepper T.T.

Directions:

1. **Cook the rotini pasta** according to the package instructions until it's al dente. Once done, drain the pasta and set it aside.
2. **While the pasta is cooking**, heat a large skillet over medium heat and add the unsalted butter. Allow it to melt and then add the minced garlic. Sauté until the garlic is fragrant, about 1 minute.
3. **Slice the yellow bell pepper** into thin strips and add it to the skillet. Sauté the bell pepper until it's tender and slightly charred.
4. **Add the spinach to the skillet.** Cook until the spinach has wilted, stirring frequently.
5. **Reduce the heat to low** and add the Vegan Miyoko's Savory Scallion Cream Cheese to the skillet. Stir until the cream cheese has melted and forms a creamy sauce with the vegetables.
6. **Stir in** the Italian seasoning, garlic powder, and onion powder, enhancing the overall flavor profile of the dish.
7. **Add the cooked pasta** to the skillet and toss until it's fully coated in the sauce. If the sauce is too thick, add some pasta water or vegetable broth to thin it out.
8. **Pour the brown butter Alfredo** sauce over the pasta and stir until everything is well combined. Season with salt and fresh cracked black pepper to taste.
9. **Serve** right away finished with fresh cracked black pepper and top with additional parmesan cheese.

How To Infuse: Add in cannabis infused tincture, cannabis oil or cannabis butter being sure to watch the overall dosage for each portion.

Pan Seared Cauliflower

Experience the exquisite blend of texture and taste in our Pan-Seared Cauliflower recipe, where perfect caramelization meets balanced, earthy flavors. A.K.A. elevated cauliflower!

Prep Time: 5 Minutes
Cook Time: 20 Minutes
Yield: 2 Servings

Infusion Options:
Cannabis Butter or Cannabis Oil

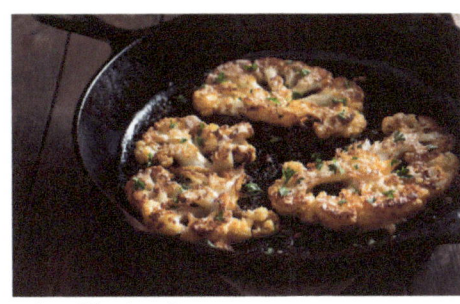

Ingredients:

- 1 large Head of Cauliflower
- 1/2 cup Milk (or plant-based milk)
- 1/2 cup Cornstarch
- 2 tablespoons grapeseed oil (for frying)
- Grated Parmesan cheese, for topping
- Salt & Fresh Cracked Black Pepper T.T.

For the Cilantro Sauce:
- 1 cup Fresh Cilantro Leaves, Packed
- 1/4 cup Plain Greek Yogurt (or vegan yogurt)
- 1 Garlic Clove, Minced
- 1 tablespoon Lime Juice
- Salt & Fresh Cracked Black Pepper T.T.

Directions:

1. **Preheat the oven.** Preheat your oven to 425°F (220°C).
2. **Prepare the cauliflower.** Trim the leaves from the cauliflower and remove the stem, leaving the core intact. Slice the cauliflower into 1-inch thick steaks, making sure to keep them intact.
3. **Flatten and sear the cauliflower.** Heat a cast-iron skillet or heavy-bottomed pan over medium-high heat. Lightly oil the skillet and place the cauliflower steaks in a single layer. Using a spatula or another heavy object, gently press down on the steaks to flatten them slightly. Sear the steaks for about 3-4 minutes on each side until they develop a golden brown crust.
4. **Coat the cauliflower steaks.** In a shallow dish, combine the milk and a pinch of salt and pepper. In another shallow dish, mix the flour or cornstarch with additional salt and pepper. Dip each cauliflower steak into the milk mixture, allowing any excess to drip off, then coat it in the seasoned flour or cornstarch, pressing gently to adhere.
5. **Shallow fry the cauliflower steaks.** In the same skillet or a separate skillet, heat the grapeseed oil over medium heat. Carefully place the coated cauliflower steaks in the hot oil. Fry them for about 3-4 minutes on each side until they become crispy and golden brown. Remove the steaks from the oil and place them on a paper towel-lined plate to drain any excess oil.
6. **Make the cilantro sauce.** In a blender or food processor, combine the cilantro leaves, Greek yogurt, minced garlic, lime juice, salt, and pepper. Blend until smooth. If needed, add a little water to achieve the desired consistency. Adjust the seasoning to taste.
7. **Serve the cauliflower steaks.** Sprinkle grated Parmesan cheese over the steaks, and drizzle them with the cilantro sauce. Garnish with additional cilantro leaves if desired.

Portobello Mushroom Burger

These Portobello mushroom burgers with sweet onion topping offer a rich and savory flavor profile, complemented by the caramelized onions and balsamic glaze.

Prep Time: 120 Minutes
Cook Time: 25 Minutes
Yield: 2 Servings

Infusion Options:
Cannabis Butter, Cannabis Honey

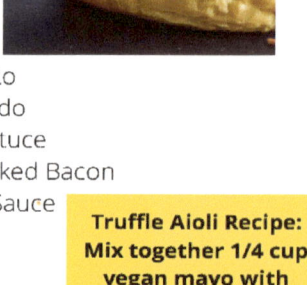

Ingredients:

For The Patty:
- 4 caps Large Portobello Mushroom
- Liquid Smoke
- Natural Vegan Beef Paste Flavoring
- Garlic Powder
- Onion Powder
- 2 Burger Buns, Toasted & Buttered

For The Sweet Onion Topping:
- 1 each Sweet Onion, Sliced
- Fresh Garlic Cloves, Diced
- Balsamic Glaze
- Pure Honey

Salt & Fresh Cracked Black Pepper T.T.

Other Toppings:
- Sliced Tomato
- Sliced Avocado
- Romaine Lettuce
- Hickory Smoked Bacon
- Truffle Aioli Sauce

Truffle Aioli Recipe: Mix together 1/4 cup vegan mayo with Authentic Truffle Oil, Truffle Salt & Black Pepper to taste.

Directions:

1. Marinate the Portobello mushrooms: In a shallow dish, combine the liquid smoke, natural vegan beef paste flavoring, garlic powder, and onion powder. Place the Portobello mushroom caps in the marinade, gill-side down. Allow them to marinate for at least 20 minutes to enhance the flavors.
2. Prepare the sweet onion topping: In a separate pan, heat some olive oil over medium heat. Add the sliced sweet onion and diced garlic cloves. Sauté until the onions are soft and caramelized. Drizzle with balsamic glaze and honey, and season with salt and fresh cracked black pepper. Stir to combine and cook for a few more minutes until the flavors meld together. Remove from heat.
3. Grill or pan-fry the Portobello mushrooms: Preheat a grill or grill pan over medium heat. Once hot, place the marinated Portobello mushrooms on the grill or pan, gill-side down. Cook for about 4-5 minutes until they start to soften and grill marks appear. Flip the mushrooms and continue grilling for another 4-5 minutes, or until they are cooked through and tender.
4. Assemble the burger: Place the grilled Portobello mushrooms on the bottom half of each toasted bun. Top with the sweet onion mixture, spreading it evenly over the mushrooms. Add any additional toppings or condiments of your choice.
5. Serve and enjoy: Place the top bun on each assembled Portobello mushroom burger. Serve them immediately while warm and enjoy!

Truffle Honey Mushroom Pasta

Absolutely anyone can make this recipe. It's perfect for a really quick lunch or dinner. Feel free to substitute the honey in this recipe for pure agave syrup if being served for strict vegans.

Prep Time: 10 Minutes
Cook Time: 30 Minutes
Yield: 4 Servings

Infusion Options:
Cannabis Butter or Cannabis Tincture or Cannabis Oil

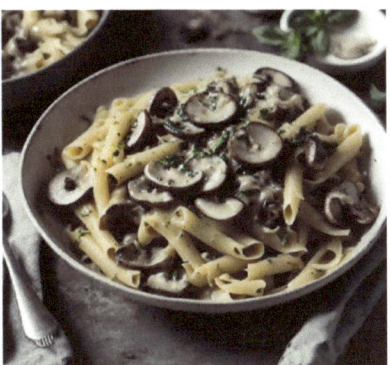

Ingredients:
- 8 ounces Baby Bella Mushroom, Sliced
- 1/2 each Sweet Onion, Diced
- 2 each Fresh Garlic Cloves, Diced
- 8 ounces Pasta
- 1 tablespoon Mushroom Powder
- 2 tablespoons Nutritional Yeast
- 4 ounces Pasta Water, From Cooked Pasta
- 2 tablespoons Unsalted Butter
- 4 tablespoons Pure Honey
- 1 tablespoon Garlic Powder

Fresh Cracked Black Pepper, Authentic Truffle Oil & Truffle Salt T.T.

Directions:
1. **Start** by heating a medium sauté pan on medium to high heat. While that is heating, add water to a stock pot with kosher salt for the pasta.
2. **Once your saute pan is hot,** add in grapeseed oil. Once your oil is ready, add in the onions and cook until they are translucent. Add in your garlic next and cook until fragrant.
3. **Next, add in your mushrooms,** mushroom powder, nutritional yeast and garlic powder.
4. **In the meantime,** your pasta water should be ready. Boil the pasta until it is al dente which means just barely undercooked. This is a chefs tip as to not end up with mushy pasta in the end. Reduce to low heat.
5. **Once your mushrooms** are nicely cooked evenly, add in honey and stir. Once your pasta is finished, drain and keep the pasta water to add to mushroom mixture. Adding pasta water creates a thickened sauce without having to make one. Use this technique for any future pasta recipes as needed.
6. **With your now ready pasta,** coat in butter and season with fresh black pepper and truffle salt.
7. **On low heat,** mix in your pasta until it is fully coated in the honey mushroom mixture.
8. **Serve right away** finished with authentic truffle oil to taste.

How To Infuse: Add in cannabis infused tincture, cannabis oil or cannabis butter being sure to watch the overall dosage for each portion.

Desserts

81	Birthday Pound Cake
82	Cinnamon Rolls
83	Fudge Brownies
84	Maple Sugar Cookies
85	Red Velvet Cookies
86	Vegan Strawberry Cheesecake

By far the sweetest chapter of this recipe book. Literally! There's so much love and adaptation put into this chapter as we have enjoyed these recipes for many years.

As always, we hope you enjoy them as well!

Birthday Pound Cake

Everyone has a birthday every single year and who doesn't love an infused birthday cake? Infuse the entire recipe for a cake or make about 2 dozen cupcakes instead. This recipe takes very few ingredients making it easy to make but it must be prepared in your stand mixer.

Prep Time: 45 Minutes
Bake Time: 45 - 60 Minutes
Yield: Standard Bundt Cake or About 2 Dozen Cupcakes

Infusion Options:
Cannabis Butter or Cannabis Oil

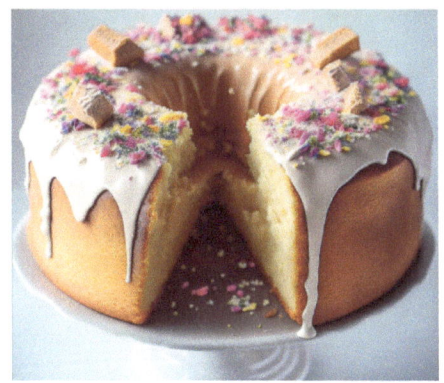

Ingredients:

- 7 Eggs, Separated
- 3 sticks Unsalted Butter, Softened
- 250 grams Cane Sugar
- 312 grams Self-Rising Flour
- 1 tablespoon Pure Vanilla Extract
- 200 grams Rainbow Sprinkles

Directions:

1. **Start** by separating the egg yolks from the egg whites.
2. **Beat** the butter, sugar and vanilla together until it's light & fluffy.
3. **Next** add in the egg yolks one at a time until well incorporated.
4. **Add** in your self-rising flour in two parts making sure to scrape the bottom in between. Place the batter to the side.
5. **Begin** whipping your egg whites until it becomes white and fluffy.
6. **Fold** the egg white mixture into the cake batter mixture BY HAND, making sure not to over mix. This step is super important, be patient.
7. **Softly** incorporate your sprinkles or omit them all together.
8. **Prepare** your bundt pan with oil making sure it is well greased or line 24 cupcake wrappers into a cupcake pan.
9. **Place** into a COLD oven. Set the oven to 325 F and bake for 45 to 60 minutes or until a toothpick comes out dry.

Variation: Make this recipe with or without the added sprinkles. Bak this recipe into a bundt cake or divide evenly into 24 cupcake liners. Infuse this recipe using our butter infusion ratio.

Cinnamon Rolls

You really have no clue of what you're missing! These cinnamon rolls are life and you won't want to buy another knock off can from the store again! Prepare this dough in your stand mixer or by hand.

Prep Time: 120 Minutes
Bake Time: 25 - 25 Minutes
Yield: 10

Infusion Options:
Cannabis Butter

Ingredients:

For The Dough:
- 3 tablespoons Unsalted Butter
- 1 packet (0.25 ounce) Instant Yeast
- 8 ounces Unsweetened Oat Milk
- 1 tablespoon Cane Sugar
- 1/4 teaspoon Salt
- 375 grams Unbleached All-Purpose Flour

For The Filling:
- 3 tablespoons Unsalted Butter
- 50 grams Dark Brown Sugar
- 1 tablespoon Ground Cinnamon

For The Icing:
- Powdered Sugar
- Unsweetened Oat Milk

Sprinkled Cinnamon and/or Icing Sugar

Directions:

1. **Dough.** Warm the milk and butter to no more 110 degrees fareinheit. Add in your sugar and yeast and stir. Let this mixture activate for 10 minutes.
2. Add in the flour in 3 parts being careful not to over mix your dough. Coat another bowl in flour and add your dough ball in. Cover with plastic wrap and set in a warm place to rise for about 1 hour, or until doubled in size.
3. On a lightly floured surface, roll out the dough into a thin rectangle (the thickness of the dough should be about 1/4-inch).
4. **Filling.** Combine the butter, sugar and cinnamon in a small bowl. Using an offset spatula, evenly cover the surface of the dough with the filling mixture.
5. Carefully roll the dough into an even log and cut into about 10 even pieces using a very sharp knife or thin thread for cleaner slices.
6. Set on top of the oven to let rise again while you preheat oven to 350 degrees Fahrenheit.
7. Once the oven is hot, bake rolls for 25-30 minutes or until slightly golden brown.
8. **Topping**. Make your glaze by whisking together your powdered sugar and milk. Evenly drizzle or dunk each cinnamon with the glaze to your liking.

Infuse this recipe using a 1/4 recipe of our butter infusion ratio.

Fudge Brownies

Everyone loves brownies, especially the infused ones. This recipe is super easy to make and we promise you'll love it! Combine in your stand mixer, food processor or mix by hand.

Prep Time: 35 Minutes
Bake Time: 18 Minutes
Yield: 14

Infusion Options:
Cannabis Butter or
Cannabis Coconut Oil

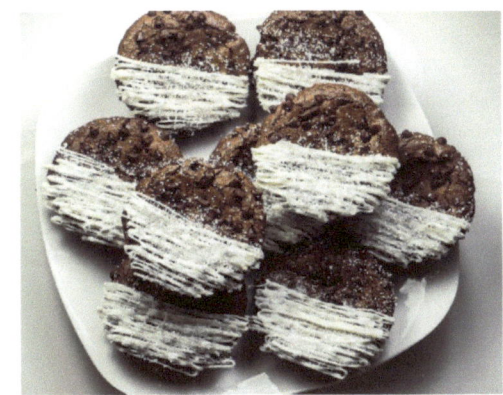

Ingredients:

- 1 stick Unsalted Butter
- 4 ounces Semi-Sweet Chocolate Chips
- 2 Large Eggs
- 7 ounces Cane Sugar
- 2 teaspoons Pure Vanilla Extract
- 40 grams Cocoa Powder
- 70 grams Unbleached All-Purpose Flour
- 40 grams Mini Semi-Sweet Chocolate Chips
- 40 grams White Chocolate Chips

Directions:

1. **Preheat** oven to 350 degrees and prepare silicone baking molds well oiled. {We prefer silicone molds for easy cleanup & measurement.}
2. **Start** by melting your 4 ounces of chocolate with your infused butter or oil. Beat in sugar once mixed has cooled some.
3. **Incorporate** vanilla & each egg one at at time. Mix in cocoa powder & all purpose flour until almost incorporated.
4. **Add** in your chocolate chips and mix until a fully incorporated brownie dough forms.
5. **Weigh** out total dough weight and divide the dough into 14 silicone cavities.
6. **Bake** for 15 to 18 minutes or until done.
7. **Drizzle** with more melted white chocolate because why not?

Variation: Feel free to use your favorite chocolate chips or get carried away and add in candy bar pieces and caramel candies. To infuse use 1/4 recipe our butter/oil infusion ratio.

Maple Sugar Cookies

You will not regret making these cookies vegan. They're so soft and yummy. No ones is gonna know. Combine in your stand mixer or food processer.

Prep Time: 35 Minutes
Bake Time: 7 - 9 Minutes
Yield: 14

Infusion Options:
Cannabis Butter or
Cannabis Coconut Oil

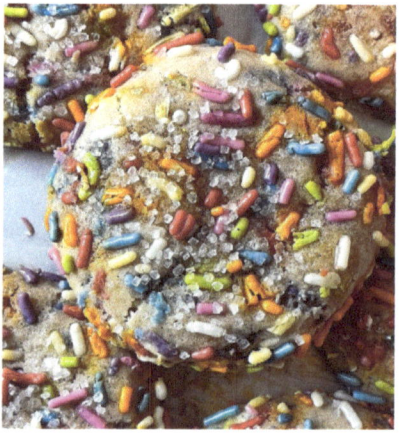

Ingredients:

- 460 grams Unbleached All-Purpose Flour
- 200 grams Dark Brown Sugar
- 3 ounces Coconut Oil
- 4 ounces Oat Milk
- 2 Egg Replacements
- 1 tablespoon Baking Powder
- 1 teaspoon Sea Salt
- 1 1/2 tablespoons Pure Maple Syrup
- 1/2 teaspoon Cinnamon
- Decorative Sugar For Coating

Directions:

1. **Preheat** oven to 350 degrees and prepare a parchment lined sheet tray.
2. **Start** by beating your oil and sugar until well incorporated. In a separate bowl, make your egg replacement mixture and then combine into the oil and sugar mixture.
3. **Add** in the milk. Here expect your mixture to look liquid-y. Don't worry it will come together.
4. **Next** add in all of your dry ingredients & blend until incorporated cookie dough forms.
5. **Weigh** out total cookie dough weight and divide all of the dough by 14. Roll into balls & then coat them completely with deco sugar. Place them 2 inches apart on the prepared tray.
6. **Bake** for 7 to 8 minutes or until done.

Variation: We've reinvented this cookie so many times. Get creative b adding in some rainbow sprinkles or switching out the cinnamon for pumpkin spice. Make these into snickerdoodles by rolling them into cinnamon sugar before baking. To infuse use 1/4 recipe our butter/oil infusion ratio.

Red Velvet Cookies

==This is the very recipe our clients know and love. It's our most popular and most sold cookie. Combine in your stand mixer or food processor.==

Prep Time: 35 Minutes
Bake Time: 7 - 9 Minutes
Yield: 14

Infusion Options:
Cannabis Butter or
Cannabis Coconut Oil

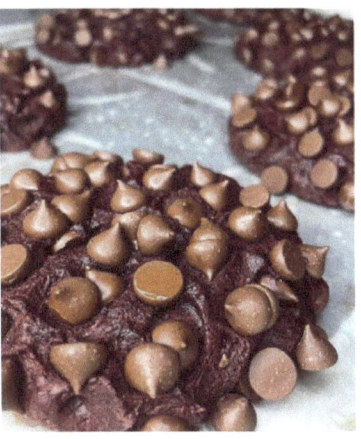

Ingredients:

- 198 grams Unbleached All-Purpose Flour
- 21 grams Cocoa Powder
- 1 teaspoon Baking Soda
- 1/4 teaspoon Sea Salt
- 1 stick Unsalted Butter
- 150 grams Dark Brown Sugar
- 50 grams Cane Sugar
- 1 tablespoon Red Food Color {Gel or Powder}
- 1 Large Egg
- 2 teaspoon Pure Vanilla Extract
- 180 grams White Chocolate Chips

Directions:

1. **Preheat** oven to 350 degrees and prepare a parchment lined sheet tray.
2. **Start** by beating your butter and sugar until light and fluffy {we do about 10 minutes. Beat in your egg, red food coloring & vanilla extract.
3. **Next** add in all of your dry ingredients & blend until just incorporated. Add in your chocolate chips and mix until a fully incorporated cookie dough forms.
4. **Weigh** out total cookie dough weight and divide all of the dough by 14. Roll into balls & place them 2 inches apart on the prepared tray.
5. **Bake** for 7 to 8 minutes or until done. Drizzle with more white chocolate because why not.

==**Variation:** You can make a classic chocolate chip cookie recipe by omitting the red food coloring & the cocoa powder. Feel free to use your favorite chocolate chips or get carried away and add in pretzel pieces and caramel candies. To infuse use 1/4 recipe our butter/oil infusion ratio.==

Vegan Strawberry Cheesecake

This recipe is a harmonious blend of velvety richness and tangy strawberries. This decadent delight is so delicious, you'll find it hard to believe it's completely vegan!

Prep Time: 1 Hour
Bake Time: 55 Minutes
Yield: 10 Slices

Infusion Option:
Cannabis Oil, Cannabis Butter, Cannabis Agave

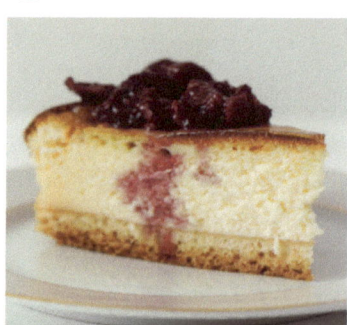

Ingredients:

For The Crust:
- 1 1/2 cups Vegan Cinnamon Graham Crackers
- 2 tablespoons Dark Brown Sugar
- 1/4 teaspoon Sea Salt
- 1 stick Unsalted Vegan Butter

For The Topping:
- Fresh Strawberries, Sliced

For The Filling:
- 1/2 cup Agave
- 16 ounces Vegan Plain Cream Cheese, by Miyoko's
- 2 teaspoon Pure Vanilla Extract
- 1 1/2 cups Unsalted Cashews, Soaked for 1 hour
- 1 cup Full-Fat Coconut Milk
- 1/4 cup Coconut Oil
- Lemon Juice & Zest, of 1 large lemon

Directions:

For the Crust:
1. **Preheat the oven.** Preheat your oven to 350°F (175°C).
2. **Prepare the crust.** In a food processor, pulse the vegan cinnamon graham crackers until they form fine crumbs. Transfer the crumbs to a mixing bowl. Add dark brown sugar and sea salt, and mix until well combined. Melt the unsalted vegan butter and pour it over the crumb mixture. Stir until evenly coated.
3. **Press the crust.** Press the crust mixture into the bottom of a greased 9-inch springform pan, spreading it evenly. Use the back of a spoon or a flat-bottomed glass to press it firmly into place.
4. **Bake the crust.** Place the pan with the crust in the preheated oven and bake for about 10 minutes, or until the crust is set and lightly golden. Remove from the oven and set aside to cool.

For the Filling:

5. **Prepare the filling.** In a blender or food processor, combine agave, vegan plain cream cheese, pure vanilla extract, soaked and drained cashews, full-fat coconut milk, coconut oil, lemon juice, and lemon zest. Blend until smooth and creamy, scraping down the sides as needed.
6. **Pour the filling.** Pour the filling mixture over the cooled crust in the springform pan, spreading it evenly with a spatula.
7. **Chill the cheesecake.** Place the cheesecake in the refrigerator and let it chill for at least 4 hours, or preferably overnight. This will allow the filling to set and firm.

For the Topping:

8. **Add fresh strawberries.** Prior to serving, arrange sliced fresh strawberries on top of the chilled cheesecake. You can arrange them in a pattern or scatter them randomly. Slice & enjoy!

Cannabis Mocktails

88	Lychee Martini
89	Smoky Mandarin Mule
90	Strawberry Cucumber Mojito
91	Spicy Pineapple Margarita

All mocktails explored and made throughout this chapter are all non-alcoholic. In other words, there is not a drop of liquor beyond this page.

Mocktails made from this chapter is for anyone looking to explore another way to infuse your lifestyle with cannabis. Whether you're at home or on-the-go, we've got you!

Make our Cannabis Mocktails in advance excluding the bubbly portion & store them bottled-airtight in the refrigerator for up to 2 weeks.

Lychee Martini

Relish this harmonious blend of lychee, lime, lavender, and ginger, crowned with sparkling cucumber water makes this mocktail a visual and flavorful delight.

Prep Time: 25 Minutes
Yield: 2 Servings

Infusion Option:
Cannabis Tincture

Ingredients:

- 1 oz lychee juice (from the can)
- 1 oz lavender simple syrup
- 1 large butterfly pea tea ice cube (prepped in advance)
- 1/4 oz ginger juice
- 1 oz lime juice
- Sparkling cucumber water (enough to top off)

Lychee fruit on a cocktail skewer or lime peel twist
Dried lavender petal garnish

The key to making this tasty non-alcoholic martini, is prepping in advance and making sure your infusion used is blended evenly into the drink.

Directions:

1. **Prepare the butterfly pea tea ice cube.** In an ice cube tray, brew a concentrated batch of butterfly pea tea and freeze it into an ice cube. This will give a beautiful blue hue to the cocktail.
2. **Chill the glass.** Prior to preparing the cocktail, chill a martini glass in the freezer or by filling it with ice and water.
3. **Muddle the butterfly pea tea ice cube.** Place the butterfly pea tea ice cube in a mixing glass or cocktail shaker. Muddle the ice cube gently using a muddler or the back of a spoon to release its color.
4. **Add the liquids.** To the muddled ice cube, add the lychee juice, lavender simple syrup, ginger juice, and lime juice. Stir or shake the mixture until well combined and chilled.
5. **Strain into the chilled glass.** Remove the ice from the chilled martini glass. Using a cocktail strainer, strain the cocktail mixture into the glass, ensuring no ice or muddled ingredients make their way into the glass.
6. **Top off with sparkling cucumber water.** Carefully pour sparkling cucumber water into the glass to top it off. The sparkling cucumber water adds a refreshing effervescence to the martini.
7. **Garnish.** Skewer a lychee fruit and place it on the rim of the glass. Sprinkle dried lavender petals on top as a garnish, adding a delicate floral aroma.
8. **Serve and enjoy.** Present the lychee martini and enjoy its delightful combination of flavors and beautiful presentation.

Notes: To make simple syrup is literally simple. You'll want to measure out equal parts water to granulated sugar and bring it to a boil. To flavor your syrup with lavender like in this recipe, simply add in dried lavender petals while the syrup is still hot but not boiling and cover it.

Smokey Mandarin Mule

==This mocktail provides a balance of fruity sweetness, tanginess, and smoky undertones, making it a refreshing and intriguing drink option. Cheers!==

Prep Time: 25 Minutes
Yield: 2 Servings

Infusion Option:
Cannabis Tincture

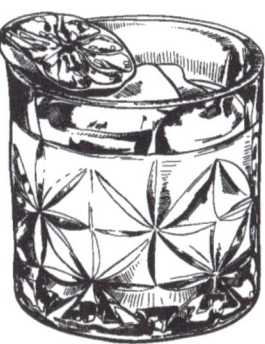

Ingredients:

- 2oz Fresh Pineapple Juice
- 1oz Fresh Simple Syrup
- 2oz Fresh Mandarin Orange Juice
- 1/4 oz Liquid Smoke
- 1oz Fresh Lime Juice
- Sparkling Ginger Beer (just enough to top of glass)

Ground Red Pepper & Smoked Salt Rim
Orange Slice or Peel Garnish

==The key to a great tasting non-alcoholic mule, is using fresh ingredients and making sure your infusion used is blended evenly into the drink.==

Directions:

1. **Rim the glass.** On a small plate, mix together ground red pepper and smoked salt. Take a glass and wet the rim with a lime or orange wedge. Dip the wet rim of the glass into the red pepper and smoked salt mixture to create a flavorful rim.
2. **Fill the glass with ice.** Fill the rimmed glass with ice cubes to keep the mocktail chilled.
3. **Prepare the mocktail mixture.** In a cocktail shaker or mixing glass, combine the fresh pineapple juice, fresh simple syrup, fresh mandarin orange juice, liquid smoke, and fresh lime juice. Add a few ice cubes to the shaker or glass.
4. **Shake or stir.** Shake the cocktail shaker vigorously for about 10 seconds or stir the mixture in the glass with a cocktail stirrer or spoon until well combined.
5. **Strain into the glass.** Using a cocktail strainer, pour the mocktail mixture from the shaker into the prepared glass, straining out the ice cubes.
6. **Top with sparkling ginger beer.** Slowly pour the sparkling ginger beer into the glass, filling it to the top. The ginger beer adds a refreshing and bubbly element to the mocktail.
7. **Garnish and serve.** Garnish the mocktail with an orange slice or peel, placing it on the rim or floating it in the drink. This adds a pop of citrus aroma and visual appeal.
8. **Enjoy.** Serve the mocktail immediately and savor the unique combination of flavors with the spicy kick of ginger beer, citrus notes, and a touch of smokiness.

Strawberry Cucumber Mojito

This virgin version of the classic mojito combines the sweetness of fresh strawberries with the crispness of cucumber and the vibrant taste of mint.

Prep Time: 35 Minutes
Yield: 2 - 4 Servings

Infusion Option:
Cannabis Tincture

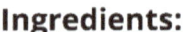

Ingredients:

- 6 fresh Strawberries, Hulled and Sliced
- 1/2 Cucumber, Peeled and Sliced
- 10-12 Fresh Mint Leaves
- Juice of 1 Lime
- 2 tablespoons Simple Syrup
- Club Soda or Sparkling Water
- Ice Cubes

Extra Mint Leaves and Strawberry Slices for garnish

The best part about a non-alcoholic mojito, is how easy it is to make. This mocktail compliments most of the recipes featured in our cookbook.

Directions:

1. **Muddle the strawberries, cucumber, and mint.** In a cocktail shaker or a sturdy glass, add the sliced strawberries, cucumber slices, and mint leaves. Use a muddler or the back of a spoon to gently mash and mix the ingredients together. This will release the flavors and juices.
2. **Add lime juice and simple syrup.** Squeeze the juice of one lime into the shaker or glass. Pour in the simple syrup. Give it a quick stir to combine the ingredients.
3. **Prepare the glasses.** Fill two glasses with ice cubes. If desired, garnish the glasses with extra mint leaves and strawberry slices.
4. **Pour and mix.** Pour the muddled mixture from the shaker or glass evenly into the prepared glasses over the ice. Fill the glasses about halfway full.
5. **Top with club soda.** Fill the rest of the glasses with club soda or sparkling water, gently stirring to mix everything together.
6. **Garnish and serve.** Add a few more mint leaves and strawberry slices on top for a decorative touch. Serve the virgin strawberry cucumber mojito immediately and enjoy its refreshing flavors!

Spicy Pineapple Margarita

Experience a taste explosion with our Jalapeño Pineapple Mocktail, where tangy citrus meets spicy jalapeño, sweetened with agave, and enhanced by a fizzy finish from the sparkling water.

Prep Time: 25 Minutes
Yield: 2 Servings

Infusion Option:
Cannabis Tincture or
Cannabis Honey/Agave

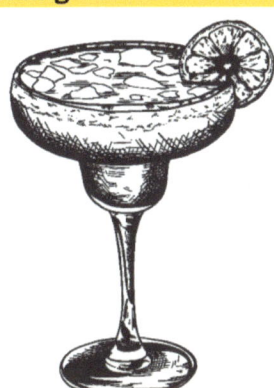

Ingredients:

- 4oz Fresh Pineapple Juice
- 1oz Pure Agave Syrup or Honey
- 1oz Fresh Lemon Juice
- 1oz Fresh Lime Juice
- 1 each Jalapeño, Sliced
- Chili Lime Salt
- Sparkling Water (just enough to top off glass)

Garnish w/ Sliced Jalapeno, Chili Lime Salt Rim & Lime Wedge Garnish

The key to a great tasting non-alcoholic margarita, is using fresh ingredients and making sure your infusion used is blended evenly into the drink.

Directions:

1. **Rim the glass.** On a small plate, pour chili lime salt. Take a glass and wet the rim with a lime or lemon wedge. Dip the wet rim of the glass into the chili lime salt to create a flavorful rim.
2. **Fill the glass with ice.** Fill the rimmed glass with ice cubes to keep the margarita chilled.
3. **Prepare the margarita mixture.** In a shaker or mixing glass, combine the fresh pineapple juice, pure agave syrup or honey, fresh lemon juice, fresh lime juice, and sliced jalapeño. Add a few ice cubes to the shaker or glass.
4. **Shake or stir.** Shake the cocktail shaker vigorously for about 10 seconds or stir the mixture in the glass with a cocktail stirrer or spoon until well combined.
5. **Strain into the glass.** Using a cocktail strainer, pour the margarita mixture from the shaker into the prepared glass, straining out the ice cubes and jalapeño slices.
6. **Top with sparkling water.** Slowly pour sparkling water into the glass, filling it to the top. The sparkling water adds a refreshing effervescence to the margarita.
7. **Garnish and serve.** Garnish the margarita with sliced jalapeños, placing them on the rim or floating them in the drink. Add a lime wedge for an additional garnish touch.
8. **Enjoy.** Serve the margarita immediately and savor the combination of sweet pineapple juice, tangy citrus flavors, and a touch of spice from the jalapeños. Cheers!

Outro

93   **Acknowledgements/Credits**
95   **How To Use Our Products**
96   **Meet The Chef's**

Thank you again for purchasing our first cannabis book! We put a lot of time, love and dedication into putting this together for you. If you'd like to learn more about us, please check out out "Meet The Chefs" page at the very end of this book.

Follow us on social media to see in action. @thehiddencreation

Acknowledgments & Credits

First and foremost, we want to express our gratitude for your investment in our debut recipe book. Our hope is that we've empowered you with the know-how to seamlessly integrate our culinary creations into your everyday routine.

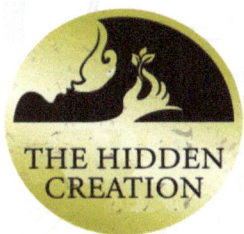

The Hidden Creation, LLC

Miami, Florida
United States of America

Email: info@thehiddencreation.com

Website: www.thehiddencreation.com

Instagram: @thehiddencreation

TikTok: @thehiddencreation

YouTube: The Hidden Creation

Acknowledgments & Credits Continued...

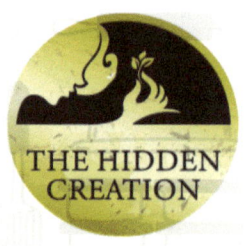

Book Cover Image:
https://studentaffairs.jhu.edu/chew/alcohol-and-other-drugs/marijuana/

Cannabinoids & Endocannabinnoid System:
https://www.chat.openai.com
https://sonapharmacy.com/what-is-the-endocannabinoid-system/

Cannabis Terpenes:
https://www.leafly.com
https://www.labeffects.com
https://www.true-blue.co
https://www.trulieve.com

Stock Photos:
https://www.canva.com
https://www.leonardo.ai

How To Use Our Products

If you've purchased any of our cooking products, thank you!! If you're out of stock or just never have tried out our products before, send us a photo of this page for a one-time discount as thank you for purchasing our book. Use our products to make infusing our recipes for your everyday lifestyle that much easier.

All-Purpose Seasoning
Italian Seasoning
Spicy Cajun Seasoning

No matter which of our seasonings you possess, each one contains 200 milligrams. The recommended serving size for our seasoning is 1 teaspoon to 1 tablespoon. As an example, 1 tablespoon will equal approximately 22 milligrams & 1 teaspoon approximately 7.4 milligrams.

Garlic & Herb Grapeseed Oil

Our garlic & herb cooking oils comes in three standard doses: 300 milligrams in the 1 ounce dropper bottle, 100 milligrams i the 2 ounces bottle & 400 milligrams in the 5 ounce bottle. Depending on which size bottle you have, you'll either start with 1 teaspoon to 1 tablespoon. Each bottle will show the exact milligram per teaspoon and tablespoon.

Butter

The entire jar is 2 ounces. You can easily get 4 to 12 doses from it. For example, 1 tablespoon gives you 25 milligrams or teaspoon gives you about 8.3 milligrams. The dosing direction will also be found on the jar.

MCT Tincture

Our tincture comes in 3 standard doses: 250 milligrams, 500 milligrams & 1000 milligrams. No matter which one you have, start with either .5 milliliter or 1 full milliliter. Each of our tincture bottles will show the exact milligram per milliliter.

Meet The Chef's

& Co-Owner's of The Hidden Creation, LLC

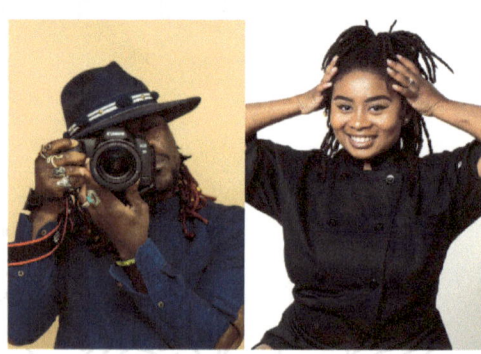

Chef Annmarie "Anna" Sparks & Chef Tarik Sparks both graduated with their Bachelors' Degrees from Johnson & Wales University located in North Miami, Florida.

PHOTO OF TARIK (LEFT) & ANNA (RIGHT)

Tarik Sparks studied for 4 years in Culinary Arts and Foods Service Management with a Concentration in Beverages. He also owns Tarik Sparks Studios where he captures elegant photography and videography of food, fashion & art. Check out his Instagram: @tariksparksstudios

Annmarie Sparks studied for 4 years in Baking & Pastry Arts and Food Service Management with a Concentration in Wedding Cakes. She's currently working in the cannabis industry and working on her second book for based on her other business: @sweet.edible.artistry

We started The Hidden Creation to provide exceptional guest experiences and knowledge through our sweet & savory culinary expertise to help others learn how to do what we do too. Our vision is to elevate your experience through infused but delicious creations. We strive to spread knowledge that infusing your lifestyle doesn't need to be difficult or horrible in taste.

We are confident that this book brings forth our shared passion for food and cannabis from our kitchen to yours. We look forward to seeing a future where cannabis is not stigmatized negatively and instead seen for it's full potential to better the lives around us.

Stay Elevated!

Your Friends,
The Hidden Creation, LLC

THE HIDDEN CREATION RECIPE BOOK

| 93 |

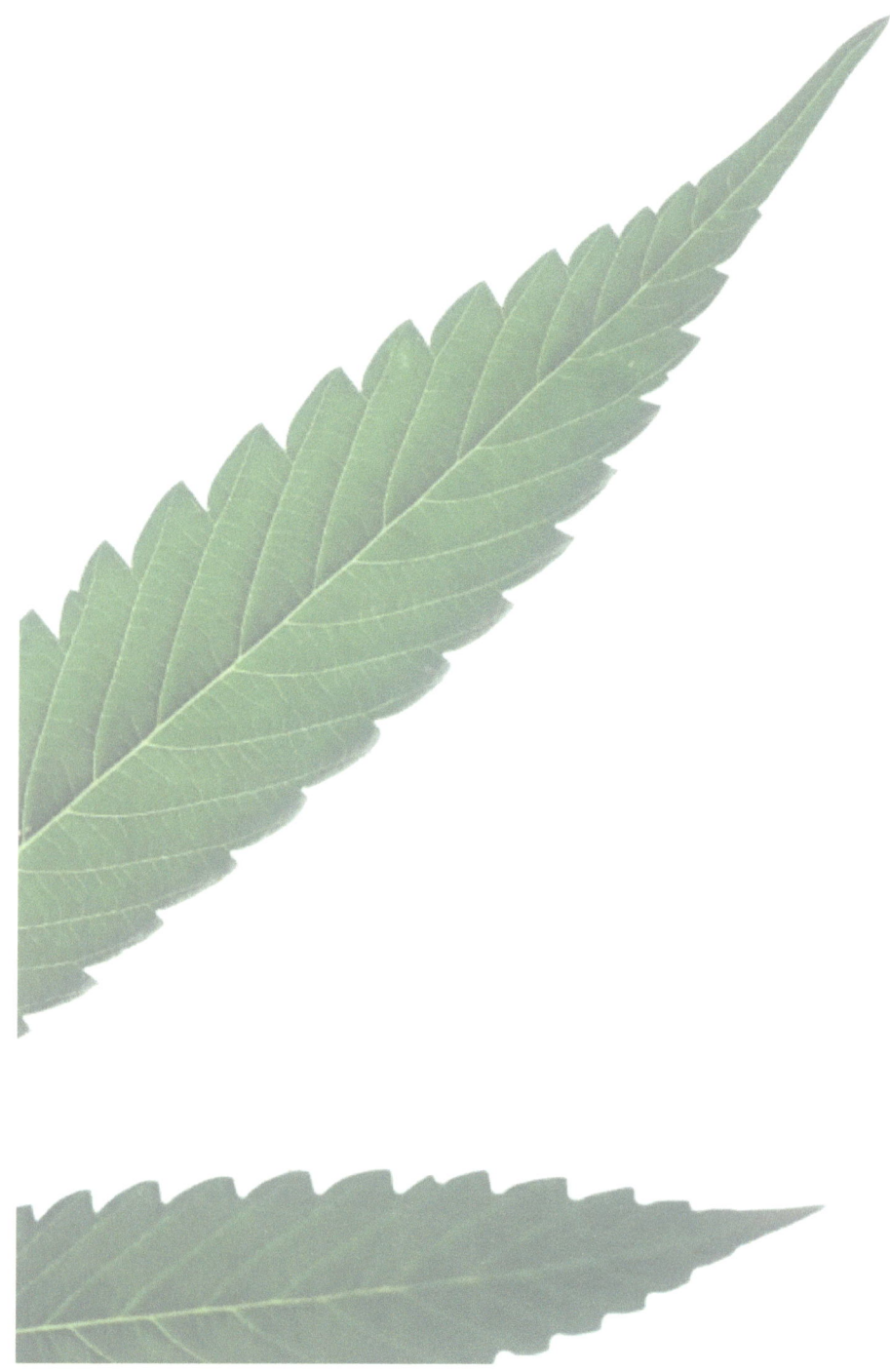

www.ingramcontent.com/pod-product-compliance
Lightning Source LLC
Chambersburg PA
CBHW041408010526
44107CB00015B/1110